Dedication

To my wonderful sons Mark and Grant and grandsons Edward and
Angus.

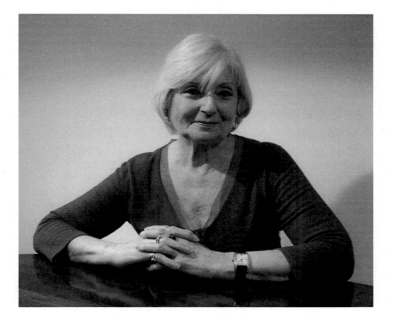

Ann Leighton was born in London where she grew up and trained to be a beauty therapist. She specialised in exercise and body massage which in 1980 led to her managing the Health Complex at The Berkeley Hotel, Knightsbridge.

But health and well-being were central to her ethos which encouraged a career change to teach students enrolled on Higher Diploma Reflexology Courses and at the same time allowed her to run her own practice.

Ann Leighton

NATURAL HEALING WITH REFLEXOLOGY

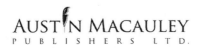
AUSTIN MACAULEY
PUBLISHERS LTD.

A CIP catalogue record for this title is available from the British Library.

At no time should prescribed medication be stopped without approval from your doctor.

ISBN 978 1 84963 699 5

www.austinmacauley.com

First Published (2015)
Austin Macauley Publishers Ltd.
25 Canada Square
Canary Wharf
London
E14 5LB

Printed and bound in Great Britain

Acknowledgments

I spent many years teaching at the Bristol School of Holistic Therapy and was constantly told by students I should write a book – now I can thank them for that. During that time I appreciated the support given to me by the International Federation of Reflexology. Also I owe a huge thank you to the many clients who've accepted reflexology as part of their life-style and have trusted me offering them healthier solutions.

INTRODUCTION

The aim of this book is to give a clear understanding to those who want to appreciate the impact reflexology has on health. For anyone not knowing anything about this subject the story must start at the very beginning. That date is 2330 BC when the ancient Egyptians practised reflexology treatments on both hands and feet. People often ask when this therapy began and are completely dumbfounded to know of its beginning thousands of years ago.

And many wonder (perhaps with scepticism) how a relationship with feet can possibly improve painful conditions. But the perspective here is that from the fourteenth century onwards it was doctors who believed pressures on feet had an effect on health. That inspirational journey continued through the centuries eventually creating reflexology as it's known today.

So imaging the Egyptians this treatment still incorporates working either on hands or feet. And these extremities are carefully mapped out in conjunction with anatomy enabling a reflexologist to treat all the body's organs and glands. The principle of reflexology is to put the body into balance creating homeostasis. This means improving the energy flow to painful areas to promote self-healing and this works allowing reflexology to treat many diverse conditions. For those suffering stress and tension – it's amazingly liberating. Sometimes early symptoms are stiff necks and headaches.

So within these chapters there's a chance to practise 'hands on' for oneself, (by working on a hand), or for family and friends who can opt to have reflexology on either hands or feet.

And for babies too there are a few simple soothing reflex massage exercises, Reflexology is an incredible science described as holistic. But what does this mean? And how does it work? These are precisely the reasons this book has been written to explain the natural process of self-healing with reflexology combined with exploring the natural properties in food that protect and improve many conditions. So even for those embarking on a reflexology course *Natural Healing with Reflexology* provides a great deal of thought provoking analysis.

Chapter One

Past and Present

Reflexology isn't a new therapy but dates back to the ancient Egyptians in 2330 BC. It's awesome to know a civilisation millennia ago was using this holistic therapy. Evidence of this was found on a wall painting decorating the tomb of Ankhmahor (the highest official after the King) found in Saqqara.

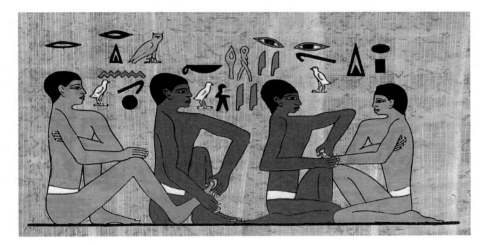

The painting depicts two therapists, each working on a patient. One practitioner is working on a foot, the other is working on a hand. Isn't it just amazing that thousands of years ago reflexology was being administered to improve health? Underneath the painting the inscription reads 'Don't hurt me', with the practitioner's reply, 'I will act so you will praise me.' The Egyptian civilisation was so well informed, but they weren't alone in believing a form of foot massage promoted good health. Generations of Native Americans also practised a form of foot pressure treatment which is still used by the Cherokee people. Other countries also pursued pressure therapy for health, including Japan and China, as well as some tribes in Africa.

But it wasn't only the eastern hemisphere investigating a connection between health and feet. In Europe a form of reflexology was practised as early as the fourteenth century. In fact a book about zone therapy was published in 1582 by Dr A'tatis and Dr Adamus enlightening readers about its effect on health. Earlier in Florence the sculptor Benvento Cellini professed to using pressures on his hands and feet to relieve pain. The word had definitely spread – or maybe this new revelation was talked about in drinking houses or over dinner because (without the media we have today) interest kept growing. In America William Crump (a steward) used a form of remedial pressure on President Garfield to reduce the extreme agony he suffered before his death in 1881. Then in London in1893 Sir James Head published a paper suggesting that stimulation on the soles of feet had an effect on the bladder. He worked closely with his colleague Sir James McKenzie to study the reaction of skin stimulation and the effect it had on different parts of the body.

So in the nineteenth century physicians were still exploring the findings of the ancient Egyptians, none more than doctor William H. Fitzgerald who was an ear, nose and throat specialist at the Boston City Hospital in America. Indeed, it was he who brought a form of reflexology to the fore in the twentieth century. In 1902 he practised in Boston for two years but then accepted a post at the London Nose and Throat Hospital, where he stayed for almost three years. Then he made an impressive move to Vienna where he assisted two eminent physicians – Professors Politzer and Chiari. They too specialised in ear, nose and throat conditions and had both written books on these problems.

However, during Dr Fitzgerald's stay in Vienna another practitioner with theories about zone therapy hit the headlines. His name was Dr d'Arsonval who practised a form of physiotherapy using reflexes. And his work caught the attention of Dr W.D. Chesney. These views were really making headlines and Chesney wrote a book called *Zone Therapy is Scientific*. It's more than a possibility it made an impact on Dr Fitzgerald; and yet again while he was in London the papers written by Sir James Head could have influenced him. Perhaps a combination of both of these things inspired him to look more closely at zone therapy. And this he did when he returned to the United States where he became the head of the Nose and Throat department at St Francis Hospital at Harford, Connecticut where he relentlessly continued his research, maintaining the concept that pressure could induce an anaesthetic state that removed pain; and that applying pressure on one area could also directly affect another part of the body.

Anyone studying reflexology today can appreciate that concept. And for that to be authentic he divided the body into ten longitudinal channels which he called zones, and that same template is still used today. However, although pressure, reflexes and zones are an integral part of reflexology Dr Fitzgerald must be acknowledged as the linchpin for its formulation, even though his early techniques were quite extraordinary. At first he worked mainly on hands and attached various devices to fingers. These consisted of all manner of things such as elastic bands, clamps and metal objects secured to the middle and tips of fingers. From this he was able to anaesthetise areas of the hand, face and jaw. This was the initiation of zone therapy, later to become reflexology. His research then turned to the feet, using similar pressures to anaesthetise different parts of the body. But he claimed that his initial discovery of numbness was an accident in a small medical procedure using a probe on mucous membrane in the nose, which gave an anaesthetic result similar to applying cocaine solution.

Certainly interest on this new health technique was spreading. In 1915 *Everybody's Magazine* published an article – 'To stop that toothache squeeze your toe' (and incidentally this does work) – but imagine how controversial it must have been at that time. This article was written by Dr Edwin Bowers who completely endorsed Dr Fitzgerald's theories. In fact in 1917 they wrote a book together entitled *Zone Therapy for Relieving Pain at Home* and later wrote a revised version.

These publications explaining this new 'science' were accepted by some doctors and dentists but did not get the approval of the medical hierarchy as a whole. Only one physician appeared enthusiastic: a doctor called Joe Selby Riley, who latterly played an important part in promoting reflexology.

In spite of many dubious criticisms Fitzgerald maintained his own conviction that zonal pressure was a decisive step to good health. In an unexpected drama he gained publicity after meeting a well-known diva at a dinner party. She told him of her anxiety that suddenly reaching high notes had become impossible – for a soprano this was catastrophic. Dr Fitzgerald took her aside, but he did not examine her throat, instead he inspected her fingers and toes. On the large right toe he found a callous. He put pressure on this for a few minutes and after release it became pain-free. Then he suggested she should attempt a high note: she did, and amazingly elevated her pitch significantly higher! What a story. It was highlighted in the press in April 1934. There is no doubt the callous was above the toenail on the throat reflex, compressing her vocal cords.

This was reflexology in its embryo form waiting to grow and develop; something envisaged by the enthusiastic doctor Joe Selby Riley. His practice was at St Petersberg, Florida where Eunice Ingham, a physiotherapist, also worked. Together they discussed Fitzgerald's theories and Eunice became obsessed.

She immediately began probing feet and carefully mapped the zones, reflexes, and glands of the body according to anatomy. She disregarded Fitzgerald's method of attaching objects to fingers and toes but instead applied pressure by using her fingers and thumbs. Soon she succeeded in getting good results from her treatments and lectured all over the United States. One clinic headed by Dr Charles Epstein acknowledged reflexology treatments were successful, but lamented they were too time-consuming to be profitable!

Eunice Ingham devoted forty years of her life to reflexology and worked until she was eighty. In that time she wrote two books, *Stories The Feet Can Tell* and *Stories Feet Have Told*. She died in 1974, aged eighty-five. But her legacy still goes on improving health and well-being. In the 1950s she trained her nephew Dwight C. Byers and together they formed the International Institute of Reflexology. Her specialised training became known as the Ingham method of reflexology, which is what all present-day treatments are based on. International Institute of Reflexology courses are taught all over the world; and for many years Dwight Byers attended seminars organised in the United Kingdom. In his book *Better Health with Foot Reflexology*, he says: 'Reflexology is constantly changing so always be prepared to accept new ideas and continue further education and practise'.

What a wise comment that was, because today we have a brilliant new concept called VRT (vertical reflex therapy) devised by Lynne Booth. Early in the 1990s Lynne held a clinic at a residential home for the elderly in Bristol. Many patients were chair-bound which changed the treatment process since it was not feasible for a patient to be propped up on a couch in a comfortable position. So Lynne adapted and knelt, pressing reflexes for wheelchair patients with their feet resting on the foot rest. This meant she was treating reflexes on the dorsal (front) of the foot, whereas with the Ingham method reflexes are treated on the plantar aspect (sole). In the same manner she treated those who could stand. VRT takes only 3–5 minutes to perform which makes it viable for elderly patients. The residents at the home responded exceptionally well to treatment, with improved mobility and reduced pain, and some were even able to discard their walking frames. Therefore VRT was born – almost by diversity because a reflexologist tried to adapt to facilitate wheelchair patients and this gave an enormous boost to painful conditions.

This is a marvellous treatment for anyone, and usually precedes the orthodox reflexology treatment. Perhaps VRT echoes the footsteps of Dr. Fitzgerald who used a probe and then realised the pressure had unintentionally caused numbness. This confirmed his belief that pressure was crucial in zone therapy.

With VRT pressure is felt more acutely due to weight bearing because the patient is standing. So these treatments feel much stronger than when a foot is treated on a patient who is lying down, because then the feet are weightless. Initially VRT was programmed to benefit skeletal problems such as neck, shoulder, hip, back and knee, but now Lynne has devised techniques that treat the body as a whole. She also introduced a synergy technique which involves patient participation to enhance recovery. It requires the patient to press the significant reflex on the hand while at the same time the reflexologist presses the corresponding reflex on the foot. The result is really worthwhile.

VRT workshops are available not only in the UK but also worldwide. The qualification gives a wider scope for treatment performance. This was my experience after training with Lynne in 1998. The first client of mine to have VRT had painful hips and understood she would feel the pressures on her feet more acutely because she was standing. However when the hip reflex was pressed she gasped loudly. *Very* loudly. It clearly demonstrated that future sessions incorporating VRT would be taboo. But when treatment ended she asked to re-book, adding she particularly wanted VRT because her hip already felt better. What a great relief! As she left she smiled, saying, 'There's no gain without pain'. So when another patient, Jane telephoned to say she'd hurt her back and couldn't stand up straight, recommending VRT was crucial. She arrived totally bent over. What followed was sensational: as the treatment progressed Jane slowly unfurled – and left walking upright! There is no doubt that combined treatments of reflexology with VRT are excellent.

This has brought the history of reflexology up to date and following its progress through the centuries one vital thread emerges: that all the investigative research was done by eminent physicians. Knowing how it was structured and developed by a medical fraternity should dismiss any doubts about the credibility of this treatment. Reflexology is a successful holistic therapy because it treats the body as a whole – relating to anatomy, not something contrived from some mystical process. Holism is based on the principle of the body's ability to self-heal. Many other therapies follow this format, including acupuncture, shiatsu and homeopathy. Similar to reflexology acupuncture sees the body divided into channels, but in acupuncture they're called meridians. And within these channels natural energy is transported around the body – and it's this natural energy that promotes healing.

Most people associate 'holistic' with health – beyond that the true essence of its meaning is relatively unknown; and yet anyone considering having treatment should be curious about its definition because it opens up an awareness on a different level of thought. It's an intriguing science that needs to be evaluated, so the following chapter sets out to explore holism from its roots, which start in Greece.

Chapter Two

Holism

To appreciate 'holistic' the word itself needs to be defined. It originates from the Greek word 'holos' which means whole and healthy. So a holistic treatment relates not only to a healthy body but encompasses the whole human factor – mind, body, spirit/soul. But what does this mean? Mind and body are easily defined, but spirit stretches our imagination because it's more elusive. It doesn't involve religion but refers to the inner self – emotions and compassion. It relates to appreciation and perceptiveness. Sometimes an awareness of spirituality can be felt listening to music or viewing art because it emanates from the soul of the artist.

Even a sunset or the natural beauty of flowers depict spirituality by their implicit simplicity and purity. Therefore spirit/soul is within all of us but not necessarily recognised, but together with mind and body it evolves into holism.

And this small word is so meaningful to health because it refers to wholeness. So a holistic treatment not only treats the whole person – mind, body and spirit – but recognises the importance of energy flow which promotes self-healing. And because reflexology treats holistically it's successful in healing many diverse conditions without causing harm. However, it is necessary to understand that reflexology cannot cure serious conditions already manifested in the body, e.g. Parkinson's disease, but it can help with side-effects, especially for cancer patients. For serious illness orthodox medicine cannot be ignored although it is believed some medication strips the body of its ability to self-heal. The principle of reflexology is its ability to put the body into homeostatis – this means a balance between all nine systems of the body. Therefore if a reflexologist finds a deviation in one system during treatment it is possible this has caused yet another system to be affected.

Putting the body back into balance means the presenting condition has been treated. Equilibrium is achieved by stimulating an underactive area and lowering an overactive area. For example during treatment someone with low blood pressure would find this raised after treatment, and high blood pressure reduced.

> A client of mine with high blood pressure used his own monitor at home after treatment and found his B.P. had lowered considerably.

But how is the body able to do this? It relates to the body's ability to self-heal. The healing process in reflexology is activated by the constant flow of energy flowing through the zones. This constant flow bathes all cells and all cells need energy to be functional. Sometimes this energy is referred to as life-force; in China it's called *chi*, in India it's called *Shakti* or *prana* and in some countries known as *aura* or *élan vital*. But what is significant is that this energy that nourishes and activates all cells promotes healing. The Chinese maintain that *chi* circulates 24 times in a day and 24 times at night.

The life-force used in oriental medicine was discovered over 4,000 years ago and it was the ancient Chinese who believed that when the mind is in turmoil then energy in the body is depleted and good health can only be restored by increasing the energy flow.

Today Ayurvedic medicine is widely used in eastern hemispheres where it is highly regarded. It treats patients holistically, that is incorporating mind, body and spirit combined with emphasis on diet for healing and reading the *aura* for diagnosis.

In 1995 D.D. Palmer, the founder of chiropractic, believed a force beyond human understanding flowed from the brain to all parts of the body and that any interference of the flow could cause disease. Similarly Samuel Hahneman, who developed homeopathy, held the same convictions about imbalances in the body. These he called miasms that originated in the life-force influencing subtle energies in the body. Homeopathy works on the principle of resonance, so that treatments involve application of the

> Hippocrates stated, 'Disease is not an entity but a fluctuating condition of the patient's body, a battle between the substances of disease and the natural self-healing tendency of the body.'

same. This in turn causes enhanced vibration in the body which then restores balance to the energy fields – the life-force then becomes more balanced, enabling the body to heal itself.

This underlines how other eminent practitioners were all embracing the same view regarding energy flow. And again this is substantiated by medical scientists today who acknowledge an energy field (life-force/*chi*) exists and enables self-healing to take place.

Physicists also agree that diseases probably occur when there is an impairment or blockage in the energy flow. But reflexology treatments are based on that fact. Reflexologists know when a reflex is pressed and feels sensitive to the patient there is congestion around that reflex. It means the energy flow is inhibited and probably stagnant throughout the zone, and this can have a knock-on effect on other reflexes located in the same zone. This is similar to plumbing.

If there's a blockage in the central heating system, more than one radiator may be affected. But in the body how can this be remedied? Once again it's down to energy flow. So the first aim of the reflexologist is to treat sensitive reflexes, and remove congestion so that the body can self-heal; the principle of holism and the main focus of this chapter.

The reason this chapter has been devoted to holism is to explain its very profound logic of seeing the body as a whole – and recognise these areas are integral in putting the body back in balance. It's such a huge concept to take on board. And yet some of the following illustrations of this are even more mind-blowing.

Quantum physicists describe the human energy field as a hologram in which every part contains information about the whole. This is very similar to DNA. But the most amazing example of this was work done by a Russian photographer, Seymion Kirlian, an electronics engineer who many decades ago developed a camera which generated a very high frequency. This had the effect of attracting rays of luminescence when focused on the human body, and it was thought he'd photographed the aura. But then plants were given the Kirlian technique. A leaf was cut in half, but when photographed was shown intact – as a **whole** leaf.

Although this was amazing, more was to follow – a hole was cut in the centre of a leaf, then when photographed it revealed the hole filled with a minute replica of the **whole** leaf. This indicates that even within plants there is an energy form that exists as a hologram in which each and every part is a blueprint of the **whole**. Perhaps this can explain the removal of phantom limb pain suffered by amputees.

The pain is real. It affects 99% of amputees who experience acute pain in a limb that no longer exists. So if a lower part of the arm is amputated pain is felt in the phantom lower arm and hand. In the United States Dr V.S. Ramachandran, an Indian-born behavioural neurologist, treats amputees using a large mirror arranged perpendicular to the patient's body. If a lower arm has been removed the patient sits with the stump at one side of the mirror and the intact arm on the other. Moving both arm and stump simultaneously gives an illusion of two intact arms. Doctor Ramachandran reported this as 'a successful amputation of a phantom limb'.

This treatment removed pain by the misconception of seeing the body complete; a blueprint of the whole. The same equation found by Kirlian using specialised photography on leaves.

Reading about Dr Ramachandran's work on amputees might seem far removed from holism. But it's not. Both the Kirlian technique that worked on energy and Dr Ramachandran's theory based on illusion created ultimately something **whole**.

'We are all inter-connected through energy – people, animals and plants. When we truly realise this, we will live with more compassion and love, our real state of being.'

Kajsa Krisha Borans, author of *Principles in Reiki*.

The reality of holism seen as wholesome and healthy is also important in eating. Dr Andrew Weil is a leading physician and health counsellor and regards himself as a mind/body practitioner. In his book *8 Weeks to Optimum Health* he says, 'The body always strives for homeostasis'. And having that balance in the body is of the upmost necessity for good health. The body's energy is fuelled by what we eat, so a lowered energy reduces the dynamics of the life-force and the body's ability to self-heal.

Hippocrates said 'Let food be your medicine and medicine your food.'

Reading about these exceptional accounts of holism must not deter from their basic concept which is simply the embodiment of mind, body and spirit. Therefore holism is an integral part of natural healing with reflexology. This amazing treatment can either be done on hands or feet. The latter are more frequently used and are also more tactile, compared with hands always open to the elements and in everyday usage. Because treatments are closely related to anatomy and physiology a reflexologist needs to know how the body works for treatments to be successful and this enables them to plan treatments for specific conditions.

So many people ask how 'massaging feet' can have any positive impact on health.

Well, firstly, reflexology is not a foot massage and a treatment works on all organs and glands in the body. However, feet come in all shapes and sizes, so the horizontal lines showing diaphragm, waistline and heel line are the

A foot has 26 bones, 21 muscles, 50 ligaments, 500 blood vessels and three distinct arches.

reflexologist's guide for accurate location. (Diagram A) The following chapter explains how reflexology works.

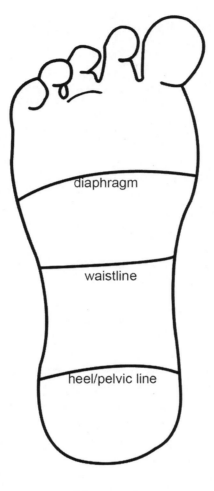

diaphragm

waistline

heel/pelvic line

Diagram A

Chapter Three

Body and Sole

In reflexology treatments the life-force/*chi* plays a key role as it flows continuously through the channels, of which there are ten. They start at the top of the head then cover the upper part of the chest where they divide so that each arm has five zones that extend one to each finger. Then these ten zones continue to the lower torso and again divide so that there are five zones in each leg, with one zone extending to each toe. (Diagram B) And within these channels are all the reflexes appertaining to anatomy together with the continuous flow of natural energy – life-force/*chi*. This combination helps to achieve homeostatis.

Viewing the diagram of the feet with all the reflexes in place does look totally bewildering, and to describe every specific detail would be too complex to follow in book form without vocational guidance. However, reading about the basic essential aspects of reflexology is both enlightening and intriguing, and will help to formulate its meaning. Every reflex represents a part of the anatomy – this fantastic structure where everything is interlinked. Our bodies have nine different systems which will be explained as treatment is defined. But the hundred dollar question is, how does reflexology work? It is of course based on treating all the reflexes shown on diagrams C & D. And to envisage feet imaging the body is difficult, but Diagram E shows how if the **head reflex** (large toes) overlap it's possible to recognise the upper part of the body. The mid-line represents the vertebral column seen on both feet which is central on the body.

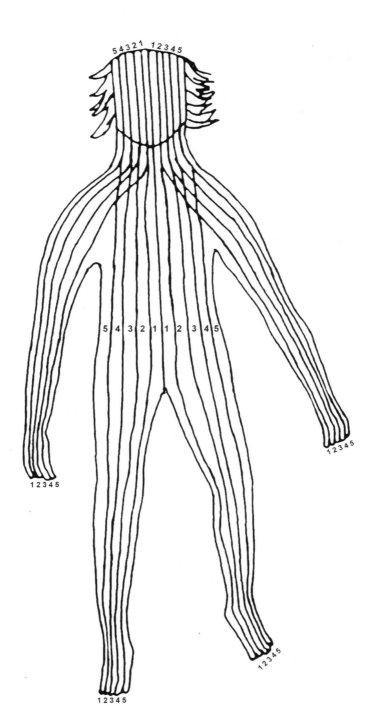

Diagram B
Ten zones of the body

Before treatment a short massage is given both for relaxation and to familiarise awareness of touch. The **head, neck** and **shoulder** reflexes are not necessarily the first to be worked in treatment. However they are in communication with four systems of the body. This makes them ideal for summarising a treatment.

These systems are the **muscular, skeletal, central nervous,** and **endocrine,** and they all perform specific functions. Muscles all over the body interact with the skeletal system to create movement. This enables the head to turn and neck to nod. Likewise shoulders are able to shrug and rotate. So one can see that the neck and shoulders are part of both **muscular** and **skeletal** systems. Also included here is the head (skull) which contains the brain – **central nervous** system. Thyroid and parathyroid glands found at the front of the neck belong to the **endocrine** system.

So how do reflexes fit in here? At the base of the large toe is the **neck** reflex. It's both at the front and back of the toe. The front relates to the throat where thyroid and parathyroid glands are found. If the **neck** reflex at the back of the large toe feels tender when pressed it could indicate stress or tension, but if the **neck** reflex at the front feels sensitive then it could relate to a sore throat; or, as in the case of the American diva written about in Chapter One, the voice box (larynx). But the thyroid gland cannot be overlooked. It has a massive impact on the body. Within its structure are four tiny parathyroid glands that regulate the calcium content in the body. Like all the other glands of the **endocrine** system it releases hormones directly into the bloodstream. One, called thyroxine, is responsible for metabolism and growth, particularly in children. If underactive, it causes tiredness, feeling cold and weight gain; if overactive, it causes thinness, anxiety and high body temperature. This gland is also associated with many female conditions. So extra work would be done on the **thyroid** reflex for someone having menstrual or menopausal symptoms. And for these problems reflexology is very beneficial. The **pituitary** reflex (seen in diagrams

> Premenstrual Syndrome
>
> In a recent study, 36 women suffering PMS were given 8 hours of therapy. 18 received bona fide reflexology. The others were given a placebo treatment. Those who received reflexology experienced a marked benefit.

C & D) at the centre of the fleshy part of the large toe is the master gland of the **endocrine** system. It's a tiny gland no larger than a pea and yet has a phenomenal task because it's able to regulate every other gland within this system. Close to the pituitary is the pineal gland which releases a hormone called melatonin. This hormone responds to changes in light, and is produced during darkness. It therefore has an effect on sleep patterns. In America melatonin tablets can be bought over the counter which helps enormously with jetlag, re-balancing the time span.

Altogether there are fourteen glands in the **endocrine** system and already six have been mentioned, but the hormones they secrete have a crucial effect on bodily functions and health. The following is just a short list of some health problems caused if hormone secretion is unbalanced and can be the reason for wanting a reflexology treatment.

Heartbeat	Infertility
Blood pressure	Impotency
Fluid retention	Hair loss
Bone loss	Anxiety
Libido	Fatigue

However, before any treatment it's necessary to have a consultation. It's so important to know a patient's full medical history, the surgery they're registered with and any medication prescribed. This is when the present condition and a reflexology programme can be discussed. Every treatment is logged, noting any reflexes showing sensitivity, tenderness or pain, and with the reflexologist's expertise a treatment plan can be arranged to relieve the condition. This can be achieved by doing extra work on a reflex far removed from where the pain is felt. For example, someone with intense back pain would also have extra treatment done not only on the **spinal** reflex but also on the **adrenal** reflex. But why, when the adrenals are not close to the spine? What is the connection between these reflexes?

This is where planning a treatment comes into play. The **adrenal** reflex is part of the **endocrine** system and secretes cortisol, a natural form of cortisone which has anti-inflammatory properties. Combining these two reflexes helps remove inflammation, allowing the back to heal because the life-force is no longer impeded. And this result is obtained without medication or manipulation – although a severe condition may need four/five treatments. But some benefit would be felt even after the first session.

But there is another area on the fleshy part of the large toe that also gives pain relief. On diagram C & D it shows the **brain** reflex. The brain, part of the **central nervous** system, could be described as a communication centre because there's a constant interchange between signals to and from the brain which help to control every part of the anatomy. It also contains a compound that has pain-relieving properties similar to morphine. They are called endorphins. So by doing extra work on the **brain** reflex endorphins can be released into the system for healing and calming. As reflexology can also be done on hands the back of the thumb can be treated to relieve a headache – and it works!

These charts also show other reflexes on the large toe. Above the **neck** reflex (at the outer edge) is the **occipital** reflex found at the base of the skull. The occipital bone provides an attachment for the large trapezius muscle that enables movement of the head, neck and shoulders. The **temporal** and **mastoid** reflexes relate to the temporal and mastoid bones at the side of the head. The temporal bone protects the delicate structures of the ear and the mastoid process has tiny air sinuses that respond with the inner ear. Strange as it may seem, treating these reflexes can prevent a condition worsening. When discomfort was felt on the **temporal** reflex by one patient she revealed she'd been unable to wear her new hearing aids because they made her ears sore. She was amazed this was picked up by reflexology.

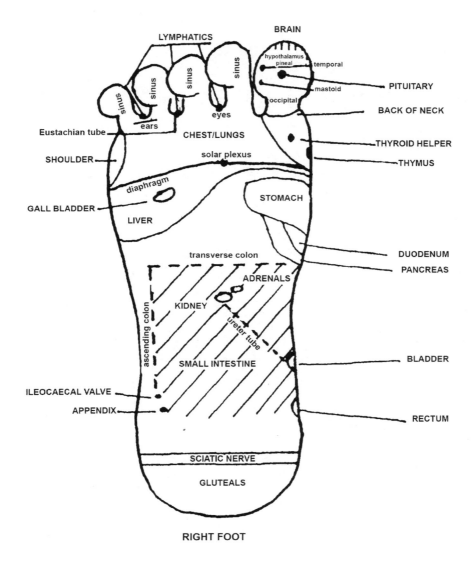

LYMPHATICS

BRAIN

hypothalamus
pineal

temporal

PITUITARY

mastoid

occipital

BACK OF NECK

sinus

sinus

sinus

sinus

eyes

ears

Eustachian tube

CHEST/LUNGS

THYROID HELPER

solar plexus

SHOULDER

THYMUS

diaphragm

STOMACH

GALL BLADDER

LIVER

transverse colon

DUODENUM

PANCREAS

ADRENALS

ascending colon

KIDNEY

ureter tube

SMALL INTESTINE

BLADDER

ILEOCAECAL VALVE

APPENDIX

RECTUM

SCIATIC NERVE

GLUTEALS

RIGHT FOOT

Diagram C

27

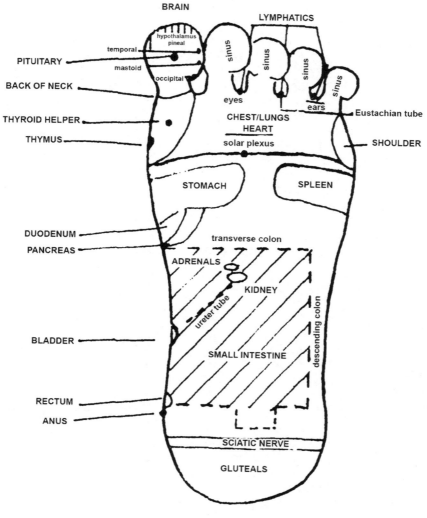

BRAIN

LYMPHATICS

hypothalamus
pineal

temporal

PITUITARY

mastoid

BACK OF NECK

occipital

THYROID HELPER

THYMUS

sinus

sinus

sinus

sinus

eyes

ears

Eustachian tube

CHEST/LUNGS
HEART

solar plexus

SHOULDER

STOMACH

SPLEEN

DUODENUM

transverse colon

PANCREAS

ADRENALS

KIDNEY

ureter tube

descending colon

BLADDER

SMALL INTESTINE

RECTUM

ANUS

SCIATIC NERVE

GLUTEALS

LEFT FOOT

Diagram D

28

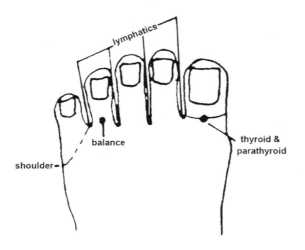

Diagram C1

The **hypothalamus** is on the large toe and is part of the forebrain. It's also linked to the pituitary. Its functions are monumental and include controlling part of the nervous system, and emotions.

Looking at diagrams C and D it can be seen the large toe is not the only digit to relate to ears because it shows both the **ear** and **eye** reflexes in between small toes; ears and eyes are part of the **special senses** system. It also indicates the reflexes for the **eustachian** and **balance**. The **balance** reflex is on the front of toe four as shown on diagram C(1). Sensitivity on the **ear** reflex may reflect a minor cause which generally improves by the end of the treatment. However, if there's discomfort on the **eustachian** reflex it's a different matter. It could suggest a blocked eustachian tube, perhaps wax, a cold or after a flight (air pressure). Sharpness felt on the **balance** reflex could indicate vertigo. This condition causes giddiness and disorientation when trying to walk. A patient may only be aware of a slight loss of balance, but would be advised to visit their doctor. Often if the **eye** reflex is tender it's due to eyestrain which a patient is aware of and say they are due for an eye test. However, this shows how these treatments provide not only a reminder but also maintenance and is why patients like to have regular monthly appointments.

The toes except large toe are also the location for the sinuses. These are channels in the facial and nasal bones and if infected cause sinusitis; and what a miserable condition this is. A sufferer not only has headaches and blocked ears but also pain at the trigeminal nerves of the face. Reflexology is a wonderful treatment for this condition. Once again it requires incorporating other reflexes from different systems of the body to achieve a good result.

Because sinusitis shows that an infection is present, stimulation of the **lymphatic** system is necessary. This system is the immune system of the body – the knight in shining armour.

Basically lymph flows through the body and has filtering stations called nodes that remove bacteria. These nodes are situated throughout the body and in-between the toes are the **lymphatic** reflexes for the neck. To successfully treat sinusitis extra work would not only be done on the throat (tonsils have lymphatic tissue) but also **ear, eustachian** and **lymphatic** reflexes. By the end of treatment mucus starts running down the throat.

This gives a good synopsis of how reflexology works in conjunction with anatomy. And already six systems of the body have been mentioned, which underlines the significance of this unusual relationship between feet and body. There are still many reflexes to explore; some will be described more briefly so that interest doesn't wane. Because this is not a text book its purpose is to enlighten the reader about this intriguing science. Therefore the next reflexes to study are those on the raised area of the foot underneath the toes. On the fleshy mound under the large toe is the **thyroid** helper, used (as implied) when the **thyroid** reflex needs extra work. At the side of this toe is the **thymus** reflex which has significance in childhood and then has little function in adulthood. The remaining area forms a ridge underneath the small toes. This is the **shoulder girdle** reflex. On the skeleton the shoulder girdle is comprised from bones, tendons and muscles. And it's this that becomes unbearably achy from stress. Below this reflex and covering the ball of the foot beneath the second and the fourth toe is the **lung** reflex. This reflex is part of the **respiratory** system where air is drawn in and out of the lungs, supplying the body with oxygen. The **shoulder** reflex (under the fifth toe) underlies the lung area. And the **chest/lung** reflex continues on the front of the foot, again imaging our own bodies. Tightness is felt here if there is a bronchial condition. Then extra work is done on the **chest/lung** reflex and nodes of the **lymphatic** system also on the front of the foot. Once, when examining a foot before treatment the whole of the **lung** reflex revealed a mass of yellowish hard skin – the patient was a heavy smoker!

The arched **diaphragm** reflex lies across the foot at the base of the **lung** reflex. In the body this too is a domed organ and assists breathing; it also separates the thoracic area from that of the abdominal capacity and again is part of the **respiratory** system. Usually the **diaphragm** reflex is worked at the beginning of a treatment. This is because of its relationship with the lungs, aiding inspiration and expiration, and because it includes the solar plexus. This is a huge junction of nerves that relate to major organs and so by initially treating the **diaphragm** it allows a patient to feel calm.

As can be seen on foot charts C and D, this reflex stretches right across the foot so it entails a specific movement for treatment. This is done by using the fleshy part of the thumb that stays in contact with the skin; so the thumb bends and presses and moves rather like a caterpillar.

Learning about the reflexes and their positioning on the body now takes on a different stance. The concept of how the body is emulated on the feet has been detailed on previous pages and is rational. Therefore it must be considered that where there are two of the same organs e.g. kidneys they are located on both feet. However sole organs such as heart, liver and spleen image the body and are either on the left or right foot.

But the bladder is a sole organ and is shown on both feet. Why? Because the bladder is situated midline on the body, (diagram E) which illustrates the feet fused together. Apart the bladder is divided showing the reflex on each foot.

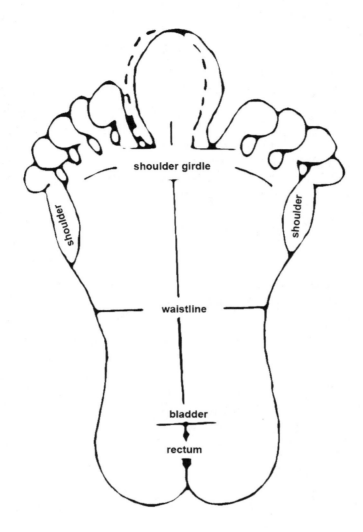

Diagram E

This emphasises the authenticity behind the charting of these reflexes.

In therapy the right foot is treated first. The reflexes previously described have been on both feet, but now the next reflexes to assess are the **liver** and **gall bladder.** And these organs are only on the right foot and are part of the **digestive** system.

The space between the diaphragm and waistline is the upper abdomen and at the outer side of the foot are the **liver** and **gall bladder** reflexes. The liver is the largest gland in the body, weighing 1–2.3kg, and has the ability to regenerate itself. It would take pages to list its functions, but here are just a few: maintaining body temperature, storing iron, aiding metabolism and detoxification. For those trying to lose weight, stimulating the **liver** reflex can help as this organ de-saturates fat. The gall bladder is attached to the liver and stores bile which aids digestion by lubricating the intestines for easier movement of chyme (partly digested food). In a reflexology treatment extra work on the liver would help anyone with anaemia or generally fatigued. Tenderness on the **gall bladder** indicates a digestive problem, or could relate to the formation of gall stones.

On the medial aspect of the right foot diagram C shows the **stomach, duodenum** and **pancreas** which all have major functions in the **digestive** system, although one small area of the pancreas called the Islets of Langerhans has a cluster of cells that belong to the **endocrine** system. These cells produce insulin but if they stop working, this leads to diabetes.

Once again, the semi-liquid (chyme) produced in the stomach facilitates movement to the duodenum, the first part of the intestine. The pancreas aids digestion by producing pancreatic juice. So who benefits from reflexology treatment on these reflexes? Anyone who has heartburn, nausea or flatulence. But extra care must be taken with diabetics.

The lower abdomen is the space between the waist line and heel line and is almost completely filled by the small intestine and colon. The anatomy of the body is astounding. There are so many components where the body's organs overlap because there's so much to amass within its structure. For example in adults the intestines extend approximately 9 metres (30 ft); so this bulk occupies most of the lower abdomen. And it's the same with reflexes on the feet, they too overlap – which is clearly evident when treating the intestines and colon because when the reflexologist walks across the foot from the waistline to the heel line both reflexes for **small intestine** and **colon** are treated simultaneously – only because they overlap. The specific treatment here is on the **small intestine** reflex. Later more emphasis is given to the **colon** reflex.

So what benefit is derived from treating the **small intestine?** Surprisingly, it helps anyone suffering anxiety and tension. Why is this? Because the alimentary tract is lined with smooth white muscle which creates peristalsis action that pushes the chyme along.

Tension affects muscles. It affects the gut – butterflies in the stomach before an exam, interview, or nervous stomach trying to cope with anxieties. Reflexology eases that tension. It also benefits IBS (irritable bowel disease), and many other gastric problems.

The **small intestine** (on the foot) extends to the heel line. From that point the dense pad of skin ending at the base of the heel contains reflexes for **lower back, gluteals** (muscles covering the buttocks) and **sciatic.** The sciatic nerve is the largest nerve in the body (2 cm wide). If this becomes inflamed the pain is agonising. The sciatic nerve originates at the lower spine and passes across each buttock, then down the back of the thigh. If severely inflamed pain is felt in lower back, hip, thigh, and sometimes in the lower leg and foot. A reflexologist treats the **sciatic** reflex at the lower leg behind the ankle (diagram 1(a)) and continues on the **sciatic** reflex across the centre of the heel pad. Then the **gluteal** reflexes are treated. Working on this area relieves pain and aids mobility. Stimulating the adrenal gland increases secretion of cortisol which (as previously mentioned) has anti-inflammatory properties.

Today so many people suffer with back problems. Is it due sometimes to the 'couch potato' syndrome? Many people, though able, never walk. And some schools have few gym or sports facilities. The body is like a machine it needs to be kept in tip-top condition, and gentle exercise keeps it maintained and healthy. The spinal column is the support structure of the body. It starts at the neck and ends at the coccyx (tail) where the bones are fused. It has 24 moveable bones (vertebrae) that give strong protection to the spinal cord which has 31 pairs of nerves – all relating to different parts of the body. And these emanate from vertebral discs. On-going communication with the brain and spinal cord is continuous as the 31 pairs of nerves connect with organs, glands and muscles all over the body. These are motor nerves that create muscle contraction and movement. But the nervous system is an immense network of different types of nerves that communicate with varying aspects of bodily functions some that happen involuntarily, such as monitoring the rate and force of the heartbeat (autonomic nervous system). However signals from the heart, brain and muscle are not continuous, they have rest periods. A muscle contraction is followed by muscle relaxation. A heartbeat too has a rest period and even a brainwave is followed by diminished action. However, unlike other electrical readings from the body, the life-force is unique because its flow is continuous. This supports the Chinese claim made over 4000 years ago and now substantiated by physicists today. This, again, is a reminder of what this book is about, the existence of natural energy in the body.

And energy is completely diminished by stress and tension and this has a tremendous effect on nerves. A little earlier, reference was made to the spinal cord and its 31 pairs of nerves, protected by the vertebral column. Reflexology is excellent for stress relief. And why? Because in treatment the reflexologist caterpillar walks up and down the **spine** reflex which has an effect on the whole **nervous** system. This means that all the following nerves are automatically treated – cervical, thoracic, lumbar, sacral and coccyx. And these nerves have a relationship with other organs and areas of the body, which creates an extensive network. All these pairs divide each side of the spinal cord.

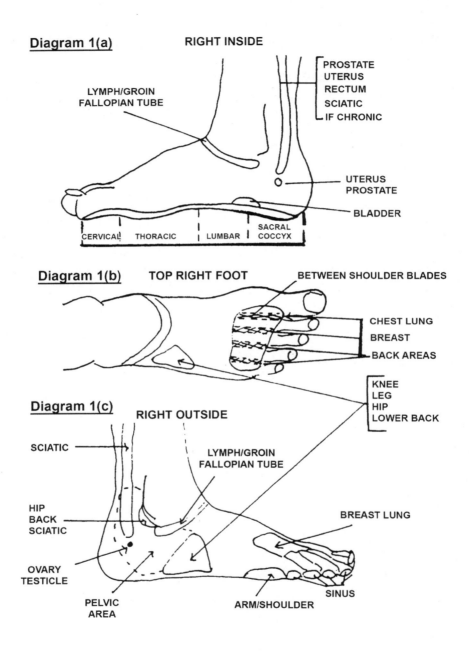

Diagram 1(a)

RIGHT INSIDE

LYMPH/GROIN
FALLOPIAN TUBE

PROSTATE
UTERUS
RECTUM
SCIATIC
IF CHRONIC

UTERUS
PROSTATE

BLADDER

CERVICAL   THORACIC   LUMBAR   SACRAL COCCYX

Diagram 1(b)

TOP RIGHT FOOT

BETWEEN SHOULDER BLADES

CHEST LUNG
BREAST
BACK AREAS

KNEE
LEG
HIP
LOWER BACK

Diagram 1(c)

RIGHT OUTSIDE

SCIATIC

LYMPH/GROIN
FALLOPIAN TUBE

HIP
BACK
SCIATIC

BREAST LUNG

OVARY
TESTICLE

PELVIC
AREA

SINUS

ARM/SHOULDER

Diagrams 1(a), (1(b), 1(c)

36

The first to the sixth pairs of cervical nerves integrate with face, ears, head and brain, the seventh pair (protected by the bony protuberance at the back of the neck) are the cervical nerves which communicate with neck and shoulder. The 12 pairs of thoracic nerves relate to the lungs, liver, kidneys, heart, hands and arms. The lower back is where most patients have back problems: this is the lumbar region which has five pairs of nerves that supply the lower part of the body and legs. The sacrum also has five pairs of nerves that react with hips and buttocks. Lastly, the coccygeal nerve influences the rectum and anus. Therefore it can be seen that extra work on the lower back is also beneficial for treating kidney problems and haemorrhoids. This clearly illustrates reflexology's aim to put the body in balance.

On the outer edge of the foot are reflexes for shoulder, elbow, arm, knee and lower back. And it could be queried why the **shoulder** reflex emerges yet again. But reflexes on the feet mirror our own bodies – which have an anterior and posterior aspect. So now the above reflexes are worked on the front of the foot (diagram 1b & 1c). The elbow is a hinge joint, a construction that allows the arm to bend. However overuse of the wrist affects tendons which causes tennis elbow. This can even happen to energetic knitters.

Does reflexology help? Yes it does. Treating the **elbow** reflex is sometimes painful but this eases when the congestion around the reflex is dispelled, once again allowing the continued flow of the electromagnetic life-force.

The **shoulder** reflex on the front of the foot has a strong allegiance with the arm, and is a very complex unit; it contains numerous fibres, tendons and muscles combining together to create movement. And treating the shoulder at the anterior aspect also includes the arm. A frozen shoulder is very painful. It causes stiffness that limits movement. For this condition **shoulder, neck, adrenal** and **lymphatic** reflexes are treated to reduce inflammation.

Similar to elbows, knees also have hinge joints. Swelling here is sometimes caused from bursitis. These small bursae are tiny sacs filled with fluid that cushion joints as a protection against friction. Swelling at the knee (bursitis), known as housemaid's knee, is caused by pressure. Osteoarthritis also affects knees. But this condition cannot be cured by reflexology; it can only give some pain relief by treating both the **knee** reflex together with the **brain** reflex to release endorphins that counteract pain.

The **hip** reflex (on both feet) is close to the ankle bone (diagram 1b). For older patients, sensitivity on this reflex may be nothing more than sitting down for long periods. But after treatment they say their hips are less stiff. Reflexology is excellent for the elderly because it's not intrusive – only socks and shoes are removed – and it also gives a boost to energy levels. For others, pain on the **hip** reflex can indicate many causes, so a few questions need to be asked to unravel the problem. Sometimes small accidents around the home are forgotten: a vigorous twist hauling something out of the car, or falling backwards onto something hard. Any of these things can trigger strained muscles, or even (yet again) bursitis. A good remedial treatment incorporates the reflexes for **hip, gluteals, sciatic, lower spine** and **adrenals** for a speedy recovery.

The **kidney** reflexes are almost at the centre of each foot and they are part of the **urinary** system of the body. They filter blood (two pints an hour) and remove toxic substances. They maintain water balance and control sodium levels, and produce urine. This is passed to the ureter tube and then stored in the bladder which is then excreted from the urethra.

The most amazing thing about the **bladder** reflex (which is on the medial aspect of the foot) is that when there's a urinary problem this reflex is pink and puffy. So even before a reflexologist presses the reflex she/he knows a problem exists – and this is proven when the patient says it's painful. Experience has sent many of my own clients with a sample to the doctor when it's been confirmed a urinary infection exists and they're put on antibiotics. The fact that this has been discovered from reflexology causes much incredulity; but this gives the treatment more authenticity. Cystitis is a common urinary infection that benefits from reflexology. A good treatment would involve all reflexes of the **urinary** and **lymphatic** system.

Surmounting each kidney is the adrenal gland part of the **endocrine** system. And these have been described earlier in treatment planning. Similar to the kidneys they also control sodium and potassium levels and water balance. They perform around fifty functions. For such small glands their impact on the body is enormous, and they secrete numerous hormones. Most recognised, perhaps, is adrenalin which prepares the body to cope in stressful situations. Because of this it's labelled 'the flight and fight' factor. This means at times of immense anger, terror or extreme excitement, these physiological changes allow the body to cope. Respiration and blood pressure increases which supplies the heart with more blood. Skeletal muscles also have increased blood supply that quickens movement in collaboration with the nervous system, which is all due to the 'flight and fight' syndrome.

Most people have experienced this adrenalin rush at some time in their lives. Perhaps the frantic rush to the airport when the motorway is at a standstill – or coping with a hospital emergency. The body feels empowered – and this is with the help of the adrenals. The emotion comes later. The **adrenal** reflex can help many conditions, particularly for anyone suffering asthma. This relates to the adrenals' effect on respiration. It also has a close relationship with the **reproduction** system.

This system has all the organs of reproduction: for women, **ovaries, uterus** and **fallopian tubes** (diagrams 1a and 1b); for men, **testicles, prostate** and **vasa deferentia** (are also shown on these diagrams together with **inguinal** reflexes (immune system). Anyone with menstrual or menopausal symptoms is helped big time from work on the reproduction system – especially for night sweats and hot flushes. For these conditions the **pituitary, thyroid** and **adrenalin** reflexes provide extra support. Again, these reflexes, together with **lumbar spine** reflex, aids fertility. This brings to mind a case history of someone who at the age of eighteen had an early menopause. This is unusual but not unheard of. Then, aged twenty-eight, she and her husband wanted a family. They'd waited over eighteen months for IVF and felt despondent. Could reflexology help? No positive answer could be given, but she wanted to have treatment. All reproduction reflexes were given an extra boost and she returned a month later for her second session. But what a revelation: she'd menstruated for the first time in ten years. It was just sensational. Then before her third appointment she telephoned to say she needed to alter the date, but confirmed she had again menstruated. Unfortunately there's no end to this story because her application for IVF materialised and she decided on this route. But this still accentuates the healing power of reflexology and its ability to put the body back into balance.

This phrase 'back into balance' at times is baffling – what does it mean? A good analogy is when an instrument does not produce the right sound – it's 'off-key'. Then someone is able to make adjustments to the strings and eventually it's in tune, re-balanced – the holistic approach in reflexology.

Another instance involving specific treatment on the **ovary** reflex occurred when a male patient said his wife had a cyst on an ovary (2 cm in diameter), and could reflexology help? Her next hospital appointment was in a month's time to discuss the appropriate treatment. Therefore it was important to have weekly reflexology therapy before that date. And this was agreed. During her first treatment, pressures on the **ovary** reflex caused a lot of discomfort, which continued throughout the evening. After the fourth treatment her hospital appointment was due; and after examination she was told the cyst no longer existed.

This story does have a happy ending. After three months I learnt she was pregnant. Any cysts within the reproduction system can cause an imbalance and sometimes prevent pregnancy.

Prostate cancer is known as the silent killer. However blood tests now can allow early diagnosis. But sensitivity on the **prostate** reflex can relate to other conditions such as an enlarged prostate, or prostatitis. This is a bacterial infection with symptoms similar to a urinary infection. If a patient feels tenderness on the **prostate** reflex there is no way a reflexologist knows *why*. The aim is to remove congestion from around this reflex to allow healing from the life-force; and at the same time stimulate other reflexes within the reproductive system to release hormones to counteract the problem. Difficulty in passing urine is a common symptom. However on the next visit if the **prostate** reflex still shows tenderness then the patient is advised to see his doctor.

Although on diagrams and reflexology charts the prostate is shown on each foot, there is only one prostate and one bladder. And again there is only one uterus. The feet represent the body, but the body is one unit. This means in reflexology the body is spread over two units – each foot. As reflexes for the prostate, bladder and uterus are on the medial side of each foot it relates to the centre of the body. This explains how one half of these organs is shown on each foot.

This chapter has tried to define the basic facts about reflexology and its affiliation with the body. However so far this has referred to reflexes only on the right foot. But reflexes for the **heart, spleen, rectum** and **anus** are located only on the left foot. This again reflects the body's image.

The heart is a major muscular organ that pumps blood around the body. It lies in the cavity between the lungs and is protected by the bony structure of the ribs. It regulates the circulatory system and carries oxygen and nourishment to all tissues essential for life. On the foot this reflex is treated on the metatarsal pad

> The heart contracts 70/80 times a minute. Also in that time approximately 5 litres of blood are pumped. Women have a slightly higher pulse rate than men.

(ball of the foot). Often patients say how remarkably soothing this area feels, even though they're unaware it is the **heart** reflex. So how can reflexology help the cardiovascular system? Firstly it automatically improves circulation; and as well as transporting oxygen and nourishment, waste is also carried in blood to the kidneys for excretion. Therefore treatment helps detoxify the body by getting rid of impurities. Often lactic and uric acid accumulates around muscles and joints, causing pain. Lactic acid, in particular, builds up if there is an insufficient supply of oxygen. Improving circulation aids elimination. Then again, it is effective for patients with high or low blood pressure – the holistic approach without medication. Statins normally prescribed for these conditions are now causing alarm after research showed many people taking them had an abnormally high level of acute kidney problems.

The next important reflex only on the left foot is the **spleen.** This is on the outer side of the foot below the **diaphragm** reflex. This organ is composed mainly from lymphatic tissue and has a close relationship with the circulatory system. The lymphatics are the immune system of the body and the **spleen** forms antibodies that protect against bacteria and infection. In the body there are thousands of lymphatic nodes. Some have already been mentioned at the neck and chest. The **inguinal** reflex represents nodes found each side of the groin (shown on Diagram 1(a)) and where a doctor examines at times of fever. Work on the **spleen** reflex is excellent for patients with low white cell count, and for those with flu symptoms, colds and sore throats.

There are now just two remaining reflexes found only on the left foot. They are **rectum** and **anus** and like the colon are part of the digestive system. This extensive system begins at the mouth and ends at the anus. Earlier it was mentioned how the enormity of amassing the body's organs and glands was achieved by overlapping. The colon is a good case in point as it's about five feet long. Treatment on this reflex starts on the right foot and extends to the left foot where it finally ends at the **anus** reflex.

Above the heel line on the right foot is the **appendix** reflex. In the body the appendix has no known function. The **ileocaecal** reflex is positioned above the **appendix.** The **ileocaecal** valve is a sphincter muscle, (circular) that encompasses the intestinal tube allowing it to open and close. When it closes it separates the small and large intestine (colon) and this regulates the flow of waste to be excreted from the body. But if this doesn't close properly toxins seep back into the small intestine. To combat this, the body over produces histamine, a problem for both sinus and migraine sufferers. The treatment of the colon starts after the **ileocaecal** has been worked. A caterpillar movement upwards is made towards the diaphragm. This is the **ascending colon** reflex. Between the diaphragm and waistline it crosses the right foot onto the left; and becomes the **transverse colon** reflex. Below the **spleen** it proceeds downwards (**descending colon**) and crosses to the medial side of the foot where both the **rectum** and **anus** reflexes are treated. The **colon** reflex is complex in its entirety. But treating this reflex is particularly beneficial for digestive problems including flatulence, diverticulitis and IBS (irritable bowel disease). Many Parkinson's disease patients have side-effects from constipation and need colonic irrigation. This again is an area where reflexology helps. Lastly treating both the **rectum** and **anus** reflexes aid the discomfort of haemorrhoids.

This now has explained all the facets of reflexology and what can be expected from treatment, which ends with a short foot massage that leaves patients blissfully euphoric. Water is then given to flush out toxins for total elimination. Unfortunately tea, coffee and alcohol are taboo for at least six hours after therapy (to avoid nausea), and preferably should not be consumed at all. The best advice is to go home and 'chill out'. Doing a large shop, heavy exertion or long drive is not recommended because reflexology has a much stronger impact than is realised. After all, the whole body, including organs, glands and central nervous system, are treated to achieve homeostasis; and healing continues for some time after.

This chapter has been solely about defining reflexology so that the co-ordination between reflexes and anatomy can be clearly understood. And it's this combination that puts the body back into balance – the principle of reflexology, homeostasis.

However, reflexology on hands cannot be overlooked. Sometimes this is a good medium for patients to practise at home for self-help. And that is what the next chapter is all about.

Chapter Four

Hand Reflexology

Hands are often used in reflexology: they are an alternative to feet. And this is seen on the painting found in an Egyptian tomb where reflexologists were working both on hands and feet. But the basic treatment is the same. The following diagrams A1 A2 B1 B2* clearly outline the reflexes imaging the body on the hand. An earlier illustration showed the life-force flowing through the body to the hands, making them a sustainable treatment for health. Feet are treated more often because they're more sensitive to touch, whereas hands are less tactile. This is because they're open to the elements, not protected by footwear, and constantly doing chores.

Nevertheless they're repeatedly used when a foot is injured with bruising, has a fungal infection or is in plaster, and treatment continues on the hand. Then again, at the end of a session a reflexologist may demonstrate how to treat a particular reflex for interim home treatment in order to enable the continuity of energy flow to assist healing. But when pressure is felt on the hand patients are amazed that it feels so strong. This confirms congestion is blocking the flow of the life-force indicating the part of the anatomy (replicated by a reflex) that is in need of nurturing. This is of course identical to a foot treatment, and the surprise at finding hand pressure strong does not indicate anything untoward – it is probably something quite banal but dreadfully irritating, for example a stiff neck. And this is where self-treatment is excellent, because when you know where to find the reflex and how to treat, it becomes very satisfying.

Therefore working on the hand for self-help starts a new dimension. It gives everyone the opportunity to practise healing with reflexology either for oneself or someone in in the family.

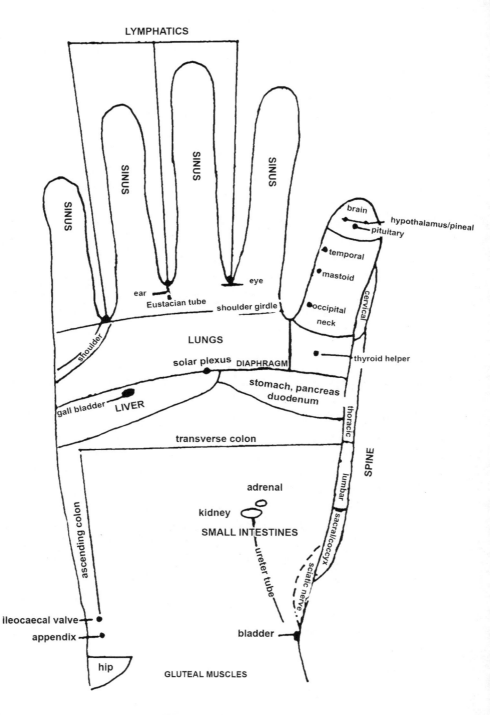

Diagram A1

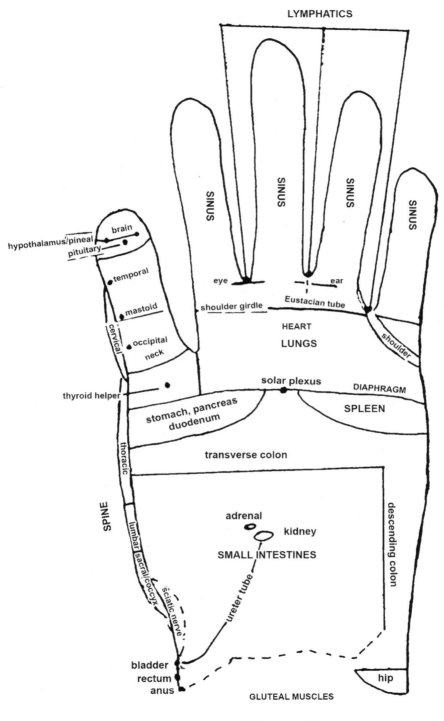

Diagram A2

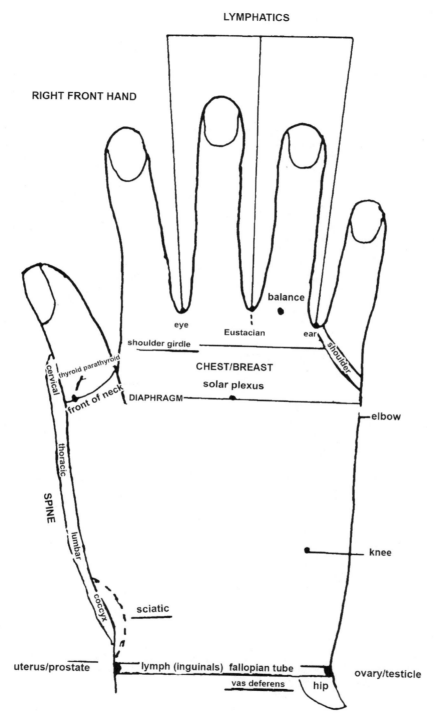

Diagram B1

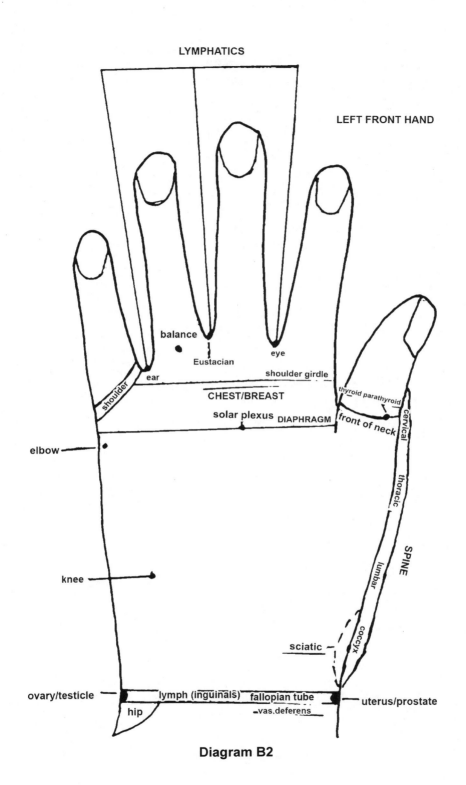

LYMPHATICS

LEFT FRONT HAND

balance

Eustacian

eye

ear

shoulder

shoulder girdle

CHEST/BREAST

solar plexus DIAPHRAGM

front of neck

thyroid parathyroid

cervical

thoracic

SPINE

lumbar

elbow

knee

sciatic

coccyx

ovary/testicle

lymph (inguinals)

fallopian tube

vas.deferens

hip

uterus/prostate

Diagram B2

47

However, these are very short uncomplicated treatments that can be practised by a novice but are still worthwhile. Sore throats, headaches or constipation can make one feel really off colour, and always happen at the worst possible time... perhaps away for a weekend when your 'get up and go' has already gone. Learning the basic technique of hand reflexology becomes easier with practice and when reflexes become familiar.

The first procedure is the caterpillar walk. The best way to describe this movement is to imagine the outer aspect of the thumb smeared with a sticky solution so that as the thumb moves, it's still in contact with the skin. Contact is never broken. This technique is used on most reflexes, although some are treated only by pressure.

Preparation

Treatment is only successful if the right technique is used. So the first thing to learn is how to 'walk the walk!' Work on the side of the hand below the wrist and practise caterpillar walking along the lower arm (diagram Fig. G). These tiny movements are called 'bites' and are made with a steady pressure using thumb or forefinger. Practise this movement on both arms, first using the thumb and then changing to forefinger. If both arms are worked, then digits from both hands are exercised. This prevents strain on finger and thumb joints, because these movements are completely different from normal daily routine. After practising, shake both hands vigorously to release tension and prevent cramp. Lastly, nails on thumbs and forefingers must be short. Otherwise discomfort felt on a reflex could be inflicted by fingernails and not the condition, so ideally all nails should be manicured and smooth.

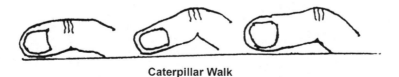

Caterpillar Walk

The treatments outlined are for minor but nonetheless irritating conditions, and it enables a beginner to remedy an ailment without medication. And if treating oneself can be done while travelling, in bed or watching television – what could be easier? If reflexology is for a family member it's particularly rewarding. To give accurate timing of treatments is difficult as this varies according to the operator, but these are only short routines taking between five and ten minutes although they shouldn't be hurried. The bites must be close together to be positive to be able to define if the reflexes feel, tender, sensitive, painful or bruised. And just to make it more confusing, if treating someone else the answer may be… 'It feels different'. However, any feedback is valuable. This determines how often treatment is needed. Reflexology is about maintaining health, so even after a small session it's advisable to drink water to eliminate toxins from the system.

Water is crucial to health and more facts are given about this in Chapter Six, 'Food for Thought'. Now for the heart of the matter – to start practising hand reflexology. The following conditions are explained with clear diagrams as an insight into self-help.

Headache, sore throat, stiff neck, sinusitis, shoulder ache, earache, backache, hip/knee pain, constipation/IBS, and stress and tension.

These are a mixture of everyday problems we've all encountered and enable a beginner to become familiar with different reflexes. And if only *one* of these exercises is constructive in reducing discomfort then it's worthwhile because it epitomises the value of reflexology. The exercises are short and gradually include the use of more reflexes, allowing progression and pre-empting the practice of foot reflexology on family and friends when more diverse treatments are explained.

Getting started. For each condition the left hand is always worked first,(if working on oneself) so working fingers are always those of the right hand. The number of bites related increase by one or two if a male is practising. Likewise when three separate walks are detailed this would increase to four on a male hand.

What causes a headache? Lots of different reasons; tiredness, stress, allergies to some foods, eyestrain, but whatever – hand reflexology is a solution. And for this Fig. 1 illustrates how to work on the thumb. This is an easy exercise, working around the head and **back of neck** reflex.

1. With front of hand facing walk around sides of thumb with forefinger five times. Fig. 1.
2. **Back of neck** reflex. With forefinger walk this reflex ten times. Fig. 2b.
3. Press RH forefinger on tip of thumb and rock finger from side to side eight times. Fig. 3.

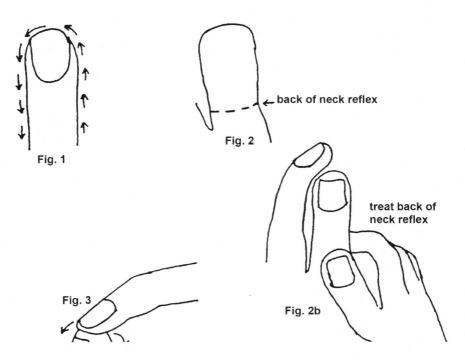

Fig. 1

back of neck reflex

Fig. 2

treat back of neck reflex

Fig. 2b

Fig. 3

Repeat this exercise on right hand. It can be repeated two to three times a day.

Sore throat. Is this the start of a cold? Many conditions start this way. Tonsils are formed from lymphoid tissue located each side of the throat and this protects the body against infection. **Lymphatic** reflexes for the neck are positioned at the webbing in between the fingers and these lymphatic nodes are part of the immune system; for a beneficial treatment these need to be stimulated. This routine works on two reflexes, **front of neck** (where the throat is located), and the **lymphatics.**

1. With front of hand facing use RH thumb and walk **front of neck** ten times. Fig. 4. Squeeze **lymphatic** reflexes in between fingers four times. Fig. 5.
2. Repeat exercise 1 and 2.

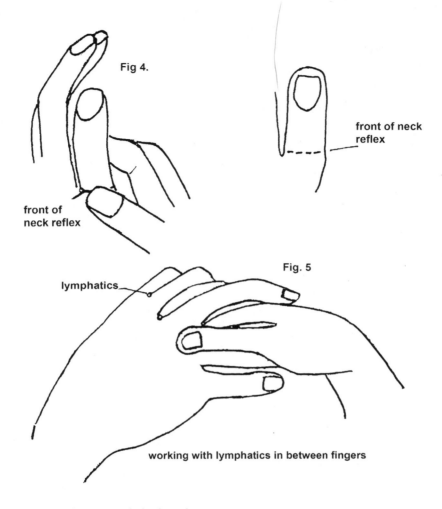

Fig 4.

front of neck reflex

front of neck reflex

lymphatics

Fig. 5

working with lymphatics in between fingers

Continue on right hand.

This can be done several times in day.

Stiff neck. – This is very uncomfortable. But what causes this? Usually it's muscular, perhaps from being in a draught or turning over in bed awkwardly. **Back of neck** reflex is at the base of the thumb on the palmar side of the hand, and if the neck is painful discomfort is also felt on the reflex.

The cervical spine is located on the outer side of the thumb just below the nail and extends to just above the thumb joint.

1. With front of hand facing use forefinger to walk **back of neck** reflex eight times. Fig.6.
2. Using RH thumb walk from top of thumb to first joint (cervical spine) eight times. Fig.7.
3. Repeat exercise 1 and 2 twice.

Continue on right hand.

This can be done several times a day.

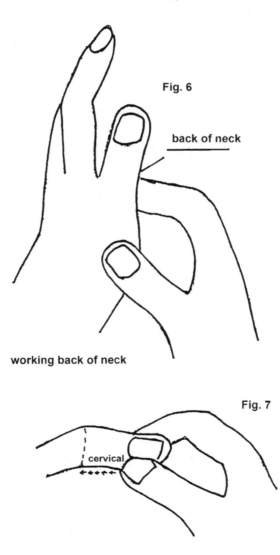

Fig. 6

back of neck

working back of neck

Fig. 7

cervical

Sinusitis. This is very stressful. It causes headaches, and face-ache from inflamed trigeminal nerves and sometimes blocked ears too, due to mucus. Can reflexology help? Yes it can. Even before a treatment finishes mucus is released and starts to trickle down the back of the throat. The **sinus** reflexes are on the palmar side of the hand on the back of the fingers and because of infection the **lymphatic** reflexes in between the fingers need to be worked too so that the immune system is stimulated. Treating the ears helps to remove any blockage or infection which might have arisen.

1. With palmar hand facing walk on all fingers. Press firmly on bulbous tips and slide off. Repeat five times. Fig. 8.
2. With thumb and forefinger squeeze **lymphatics** on the webbing. Fig. 9.

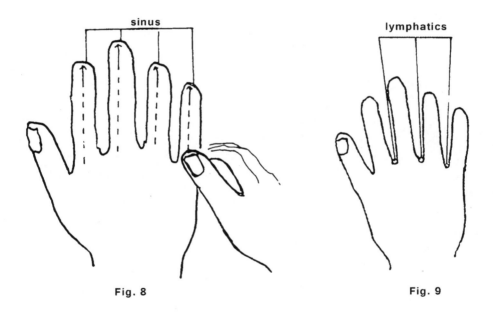

Fig. 8   Fig. 9

Repeat four times.

3. Walk **ear** reflex between fingers 4 and 5. Fig.10.

4. Then make three circular pressures on **ear point.** Fig.11.

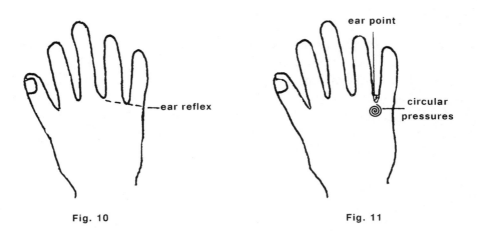

Fig. 10   Fig. 11

Repeat twice.
Continue on right hand.
This can be done several times a day.

Shoulder ache. This is thoroughly tiresome. It is usually caused by lifting. Although it can occur just turning over in bed. The shoulder is very complex: a structure composed of tendons, muscles and ligaments. If painful, it needs treatment three or four times a day for at least a week. The **shoulder** reflex is on the palmar hand at the groove between the small and fourth finger, while the **shoulder girdle** stretches across the padded area at the base of all fingers.

1. Squeeze **shoulder** reflex with RH finger and thumb on both palmar and front of hand and in unison with a slight lifting movement work down the groove five times. Fig. 12a and 12b.
2. Caterpillar walk across **shoulder girdle** five times. Fig.13.
3. Repeat twice.

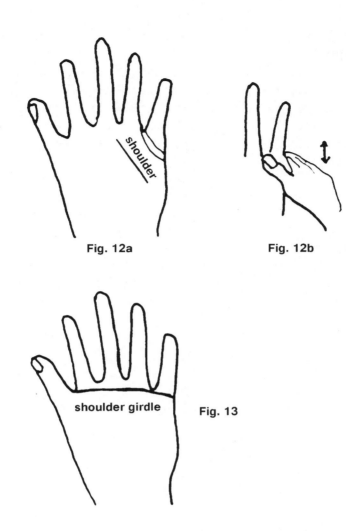

Fig. 12a   Fig. 12b

shoulder girdle   Fig. 13

Pressures must be firm and can be done several times a day.

Earache. This can be caused from inflammation or infection. Hand reflexology can reduce pain, but if this persists a doctor's advice is necessary. There are four reflexes relating to ears. The **ear** reflex straddles the base of fingers four and five on palmar hand. While the **ear point** is at the crease of fingers four and five; and it can feel very painful when pressed. The **eustachian** reflex lies in the groove between fingers three and four. This tube is where blockages occur. Lastly, the **balance** reflex is on the front of the hand at the base of fourth finger.

1. With palmar hand facing walk four times across **ear** reflex using thumb. Fig. 14.
2. At **ear point** make six tiny circular presses with thumb. Fig. 15.
3. Place forefinger and thumb between third and fourth finger just below knuckles, squeeze together gently and slide upwards. This is the **Eustachian** reflex. Repeat twice. Fig. 16.
4. On front of hand press **balance** at base of fourth finger three times. Fig. 17.
5. Only repeat routine twice in a day.

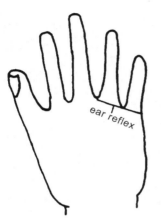

Fig. 14

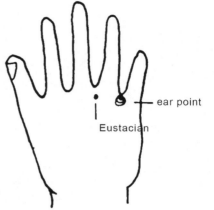

Fig. 15

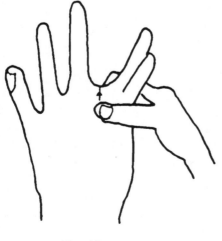

Fig. 16

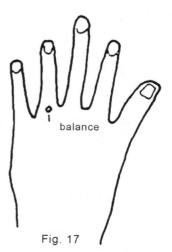

Fig. 17

Complete on right hand.

Backache. This is immensely painful and affects many movements. To treat successfully on the hand, pressures must be strong. The spine is divided into cervical, thoracic, lumbar, sacral and coccyx. Walking down the **spine** reflex from the top of thumb will locate (by sensitivity) the area that's tense. And this becomes more noticeable on either left or right hand, pin-pointing the area of stress in the body.

1. At base of thumbnail walk **spine** reflex to wrist, then back again to thumb. Repeat three times. Fig. 18.
2. Treat most sensitive area, walking across **spine** in three lines each with three bites. Repeat four times. Increase bites on a male hand. Fig. 19.
3. Repeat this exercise twice and then at least four times a day.
4. Continue on right hand.

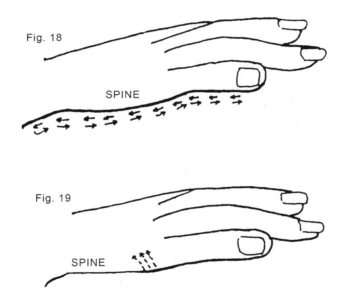

Fig. 18

SPINE

Fig. 19

SPINE

Hip and knee pain. These conditions don't always go together, but often do. However, directions for one or the other is easy to follow. Pain in hip and knee is often due to arthritis. Sadly, reflexology can't cure any disease that's already manifested in the body, but it can ease pain and reduce inflammation. Reflexes for **hip** and **knee** are found on the outer side of the front of the hand. **Gluteal** muscles form the buttocks and are located on the palmar hand just above the wrist.

1. With forefinger walk six bites from base of small finger, swivel finger onto front of hand and walk three bites onto the **knee** reflex. Fig. 20.
2. With forefinger make four firm circular presses on the **knee.** Fig. 20A.
3. Slide forefinger back to edge and walk to **hip**. Fig. 20B
4. Walk three bites across **hip** reflex close to wrist bone and repeat three times. Fig. 20C.
5. With palmar hand facing work on **gluteal** reflex. Start at latter side of palm and work upwards in lines of four bites. Do not work on fleshy mound below thumb. Fig. 21.

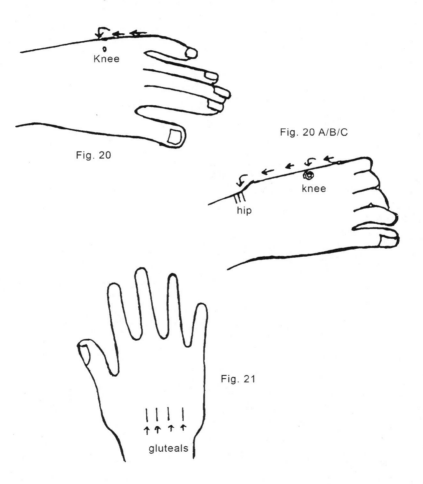

Knee

Fig. 20

Fig. 20 A/B/C

hip

knee

Fig. 21

gluteals

Continue on right hand.

This routine can be done several times a day.

Constipation. This is often suffered by Parkinson's disease patients but can affect anyone with an uncomfortable bloat. Back to the waterfront – because this can be caused by lack of fluid, or not enough fibre in the diet. On the hand it's improved by treating the **intestines** reflex. When the palmar hand has fingers curled the palm forms a small depression and this is where the **intestines** are treated.

1. With palmar hand facing make ten circles on **intestines** with RH thumb. Fig. 22.
2. Walk four lines of three bites over **intestines**, avoiding fleshy mound underneath thumb. Fig. 23.

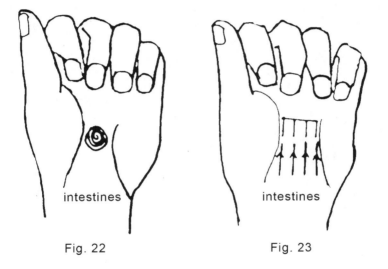

intestines   intestines

Fig. 22   Fig. 23

Repeat twice.
Continue on right hand.
Can be done three times a day

Stress and tension. This is caused by anxiety and perpetual worry – maybe health, finance, work-related or marital issues. In today's climate the list is never-ending. Reflexology is especially beneficial for these issues because its whole entity is mind, body and spirit which is reflected in emotions. Treatment on the hand is helpful and relaxing, but on the feet the impact is more consuming, possibly because of the positioning of the body. Therefore a self-help hand routine has a better effect when lying down. This could work with a morning and night-time session and if very stressed an extra routine in the day, sitting down.

This is a particularly good treatment left until last because most reflexes are already known – except the **diaphragm** and **solar plexus**. These reflexes are crucial for easing tension together with **spine, neck, shoulder,** and **shoulder girdle** reflexes.

1. With palmar hand facing, use thumb to walk **diaphragm.** Start on the diagonal line below small finger. Press three times below third finger on **solar plexus**. Continue to walk across diaphragm. Fig. 24.
2. With forefinger, walk **back of neck** five times. Fig. 25.
3. With palmar hand facing, work groove of **shoulder** reflex using thumb and forefinger together each side at base of small finger. With a lifting movement work down groove five times. Fig. 26.
4. Using thumb, with firm pressures walk across **shoulder girdle** five times. Fig. 27.
5. Using thumb, walk down the **spine** reflex then at base change direction and walk back. Repeat these two movements three times. Fig. 28.

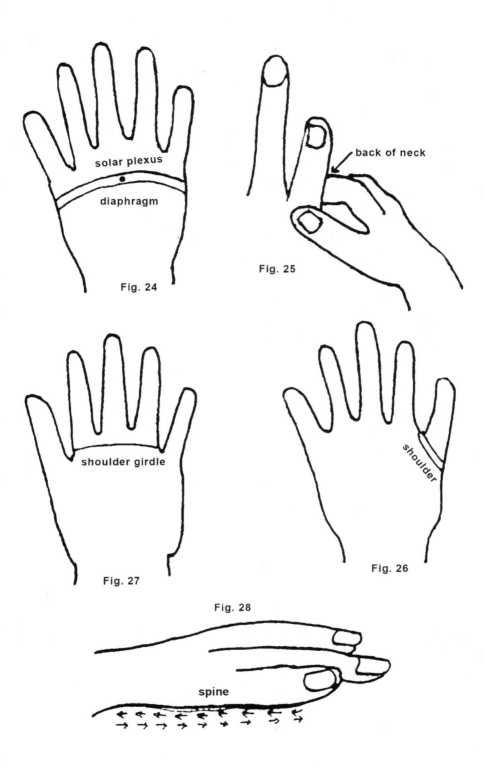

solar plexus

diaphragm

Fig. 24

back of neck

Fig. 25

shoulder girdle

Fig. 27

shoulder

Fig. 26

Fig. 28

spine

Before commencing right hand take three deep breaths.
Repeat after right hand is treated.

By the time treatment on stress and tension has been accomplished, fingers and thumbs become more flexible. And if caterpillar walks are made in a firm smooth movement it creates a continuous flow – almost rhythmic. This makes the treatment more positive.

Again, this firm technique must be used when making pressures, and in circles because the purpose is to remove congestion built-up around a reflex – reflecting where in the body there's discomfort. If pressure is reduced because the reflex feels painful when touched, then healing takes longer to accomplish. In such an instance, work on the next reflex, then after a break the painful reflex will feel less tense and treatment can continue.

Practising on hands is a good starting point because the next chapter explains foot reflexology for friends and family.

Chapter Five

Rescue Package for Friends and Family

Foot reflexology has a greater impact on the body than can be imagined. And for a beginner, some reflexes are easier to find on feet because on the hand (which is a smaller extremity) more reflexes overlap. But feet tell amazing stories. Sometimes a tiny patch of hard skin seen on an unusual area signifies protection; as in the case of a lady with this on her **thyroid** reflex, and yes she had an under-active thyroid condition. However the most common give-away is seeing a **bladder** reflex pink and puffy, denoting de-hydration or infection. So treating feet with reflexology is not only inspirational but also informative. A clear communication between body and sole.

Finding family or friends to participate in treatment should not be a problem – they'll just love it. Even without a specific condition it gives comfort. In today's climate life is a challenge and everyone needs a little TLC. That's why the first treatment is for an energy boost, good for all the family; and an opportunity to learn more about reflexology.

But first it's necessary to think about preparation. An important factor in these treatments is eye contact. For some reason it's deemed commendable to be stoic. So when a reflex feels painful (picked up by the operator because it feels crunchy), no feedback is forthcoming – but the eyes tell all. But feedback is necessary for the treatment to be objective, and planned treatment areas must be comfortable for both patient and operator. At home this can be accomplished in three different ways. The patient can sit in an armchair with the operator sitting in front on a stool; this means feet are placed on the operator's lap and the stool must be the right height to be comfortable, but it can be done. Alternatively, a settee works well, with patient's feet resting on the arm and a pile of cushions placed midway to create a backrest. This same effect can be achieved using a bed with the patient's feet at the base and a mound of pillows halfway to support the back; this allows the operator to sit and treat with ease. The other major issue, as in a clinic, is that reflexology must be done in a peaceful atmosphere, without interruptions: not only for whoever is receiving treatment but for the operator concentrating on something very new. And of course hygiene must be considered. A small towel should be put over the arm of a settee and again on the operator's lap when using chair and stool method. At the end of a bed place feet on a clean towel. Friends and family are cherished – but not always their feet!

Have at the ready on a small table either witch hazel, surgical spirit or cologne that can be applied with cotton wool if feet have not been washed. Carefully look in between toes for athlete's foot (described in footnotes). This infection is easily picked up at gyms and swimming pools but is contagious and can infect fingernails. Should this be prevalent, defer until the infection is cleared. Verrucae are also contagious but if covered with plaster the foot can be treated; or if the verruca is on a specific reflex, this is when a reflexologist should revert back to hand reflexology to ensure treatment is completed. But what is most important is: always wash hands before and after treatment.

Mostly feet are accepted without any particular bias. But those of men are in much better condition than their female counterparts. Why? Because they wear socks that prevent the trauma of friction that causes hard skin, and their feet are never cramped into fashionable high-heeled shoes – so enticing, but they are *killers!* And this becomes evident when working on family and friends: it's females who suffer more from bunions and hammertoes resulting from over-tight shoes. However, these are common conditions not contra-indicated to reflexology. If a bunion is inflamed, causing pain, then continue by treating the hand. That's why practising on the hand first is important.

Sometimes people hesitate to have reflexology because their feet are ticklish. However, the firmness of movement removes any likelihood of 'touchy feely' irritation. In fact, before a treatment begins each foot is gently held and then rotated three times in alternate directions. This simple exercise provides an introduction to the reflexologist's hands which helps dispel any concerns that may have existed. Fig. B & C.

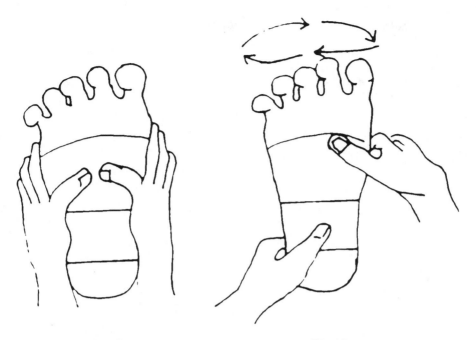

Fig. B   **Fig. C**

The treatments included in this chapter are small treatments adapted for a beginner. One for **energy boosting** is a good introduction to feet, followed by **gout, urine infection, menopause, IBS, tonsillitis, sciatica** and **chronic back pain**. Also included are three small routines for babies suffering **colic, teething** and **common cold.** All these treatments give the opportunity to learn new reflexes. To find these more accurately, the foot is divided into three sections – diaphragm line, waistline and heel line, as seen on Fig. A. The foot charts C and D showing all the reflexes can be seen in Chapter Three.

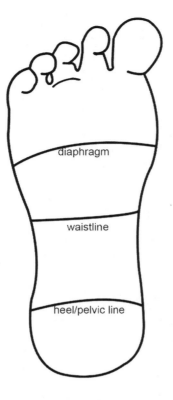

diaphragm

waistline

heel/pelvic line

Fig. A

In foot reflexology the <u>right foot </u>is always worked first. The techniques are the same as practised on the hand. Again on a male foot the number of caterpillar walks need to be increased. To be specific without knowledge of size is difficult, so a lower and higher gauge is included in instructions.

<u>Treatment for energy boosting.</u> This is good for those times when the body feels drained. It's when the mind and body are in overdrive – a constant pressure when it's difficult even to relax. The **diaphragm** and **solar plexus** help alleviate stress, as seen with hand reflexology. When the body is tense, many systems are affected. Therefore, other reflexes used in this routine are **pituitary, head, liver, spine, kidneys, adrenals** and **small intestines.**

<u>Before starting any treatment</u>: encompass and hold foot with both hands for ten seconds. Rotate foot three times clockwise, then in

reverse directions, as shown in fig. B & C on page 65. All treatments start on right foot which is supported by non-working hand. The thumb is always used to treat unless stated otherwise.

Energy boosting routine

1. Walk **diaphragm** and press three times on **solar plexus** finishing below small toe. Diagram 1.

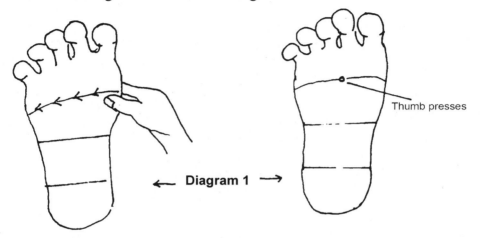

Thumb presses

← **Diagram 1** →

2. Make three presses on **pituitary** reflex. Diagram 2…

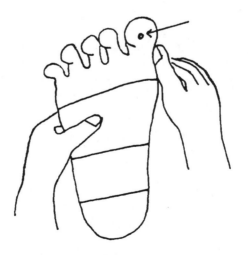

Diagram 2

3. Walk **back of neck** reflex three times. Then walk around **head** reflex in four to six separate walks. Diagrams 3a & 3b.

Diagram 3a   **Diagram 3b**

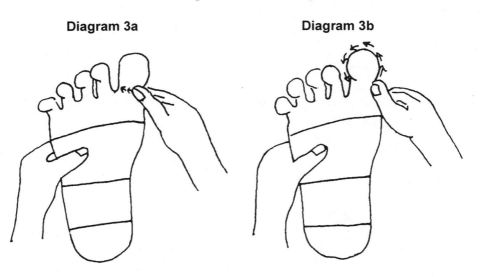

4. Walk **liver** reflex six to eight bites three times. Diagram 4. <u>Liver reflex</u> is only on right foot.

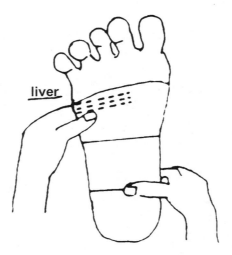

<u>liver</u>

Diagram 4

5. Walk **spine** from just below toe nail to base of heel. Change direction and walk back. Repeat twice. Diagram 5.

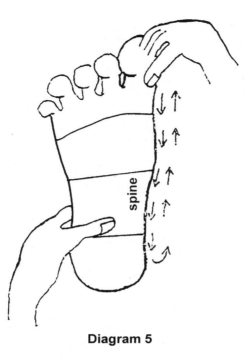

Diagram 5

6. Make three medium light presses on **kidney** reflex. Diagram 6.

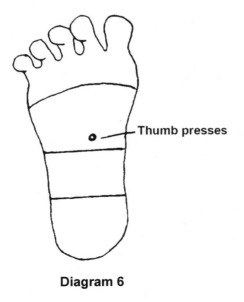

Thumb presses

Diagram 6

7. Make three pressure circles on **adrenals.** Diagram 7.

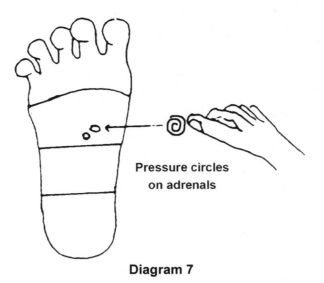

Pressure circles
on adrenals

Diagram 7

8. Walk across **intestines** ten to twelve bites. This is a large area working downwards from waistline to heel line. To be done once only. Diagram 8.

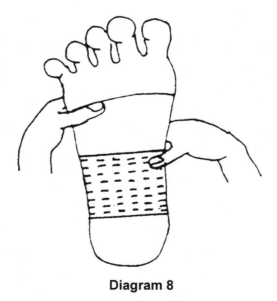

Diagram 8

9. Finish by walking **diaphragm** reflex. Then rotate foot twice in alternate directions. Diagram 9.

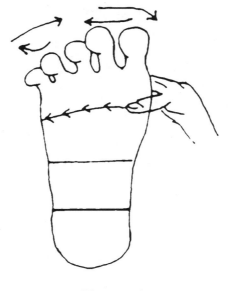

Diagram 9

Repeat on left foot, omitting **liver** reflex.
Always offer a glass of water after each treatment.

Gout The next treatment is for gout which is caused when there's an excess of uric acid in the bloodstream. Gout is usually identified with pain and swelling at the large toe joint but it can also affect knees and elbows. It is a form of arthritis when diet has to be considered. This means restricting consumption of red meat and dairy products, especially cheese and acidic fruits such as rhubarb. Increasing water intake is essential. With this condition kidneys can be affected as they're responsible for the filtration of waste in the body. For this exercise **lymphatics** of the groin are treated as well as the urinary tract.
Unless otherwise stated thumbs are always used throughout these exercises.

1. Walk the **diaphragm** and make three presses on **solar plexus.** Diagram 1.

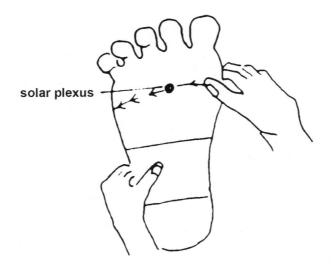

solar plexus

Diagram 1

2. Make three light presses on **kidney** reflex. Release (1 second) and repeat. Diagram 2.

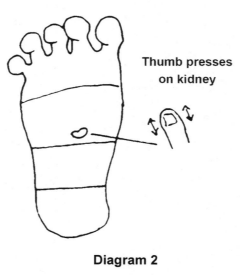

Thumb presses
on kidney

Diagram 2

3. Make three pressure circles on **adrenal** reflex. Diagram 3.

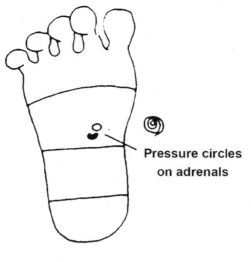

**Pressure circles
on adrenals**

Diagram 3

4. Return to **kidney** and walk **ureter** reflex to **bladder.** Diagram
4.

Diagram 4

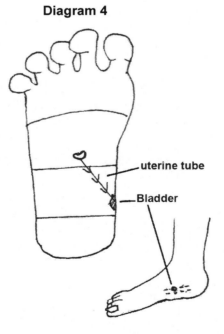

uterine tube

Bladder

Diagram 5

5. Walk across **bladder** reflex in three lines of four to five bites. If this reflex is pink and puffy and tender when touched repeat this exercise at end of routine. Diagram 5.

6. Walk across **lymphatics** (groin) three times using forefinger. Diagram 6.

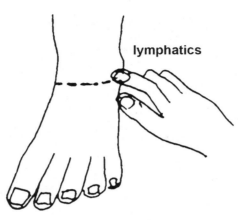

Diagram 6

Treat left foot.

Urine infection Urine infection is very uncomfortable, although some organisms can exist in the bladder without symptoms. This often happens with the elderly who may appear forgetful and have moments of dizziness. During treatment, if the urinary reflexes – **kidneys, ureter** and **bladder** – show tenderness, it underlines the possibility of an infection. Increasing the amount of water consumption is imperative.

1 Make three presses on **kidney** reflex. If painful, repeat at end of routine. Diagram 1.

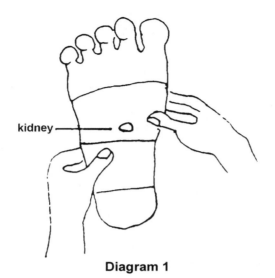

Diagram 1

2. Walk **ureter** reflex from **kidney** to **bladder** – ten to twelve bites. Diagram 2.

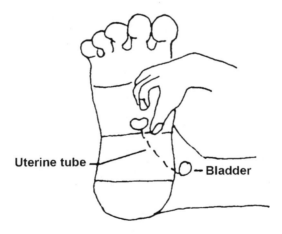

Diagram 2

3. Walk across **bladder** reflex in three lines three to four bites. Diagram 3.

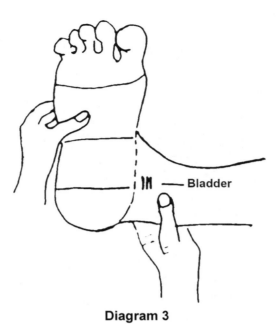

Diagram 3

4. Use forefinger to walk **lymphatics** (groin) three times nine to twelve bites. Diagram 4.

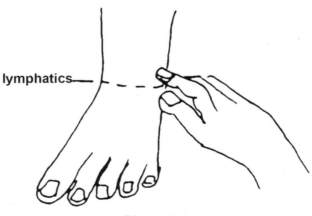

Diagram 4

Repeat on left foot.

Treatment for menopause Reflexology is excellent for menopausal and menstrual problems. It helps reduce hot flushes and night sweats. The treatment incorporates working on glands of the endocrine system. These glands release hormones into the bloodstream.

1. Walk **diaphragm** and give three presses on **solar plexus.** Diagram 1.

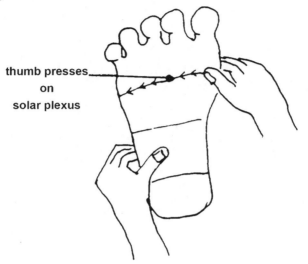

Diagram 1

2. Make three pressure circles on **pituitary** reflex. Diagram 2.

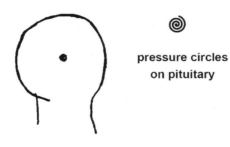

Diagram 2

3. With forefinger, make three walks of four to five bites on **thyroid** and three pressure circles on **thyroid helper** reflex. Diagram 3.

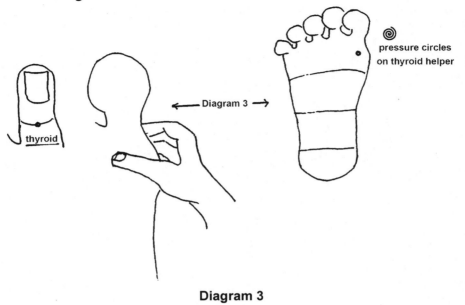

Diagram 3

4. Make three pressure circles on **ovary** reflex. Diagram 4.

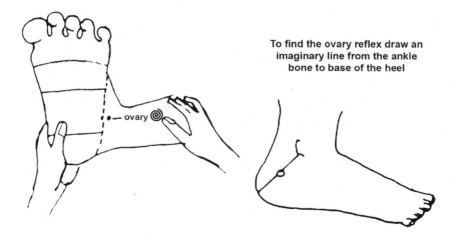

Diagram 4

5. From waistline, caterpillar walk down **spine** reflex to heel line. Repeat four times. Diagram 5.

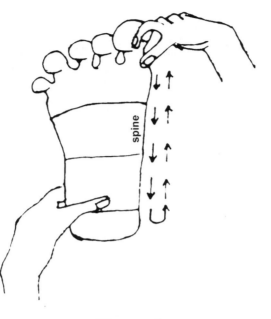

Diagram 5

Repeat on left foot.

Treatment for IBS (Irritable Bowel Syndrome) The specific cause of IBS is unknown. It affects the small intestines and colon and because of this was linked with the hand routine for constipation. IBS is invariably aggravated by stress, eating habits and bowel movements that alternate between constipation and diarrhoea.

1. Walk across **diaphragm** and press **solar plexus** three times. Diagram 1.

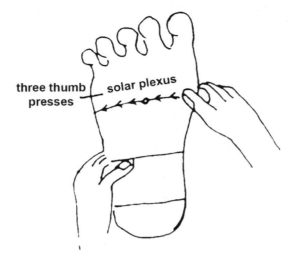

Diagram 1

2. Walk across **liver** reflex in three to four lines of six to eight bites. Diagram 2.

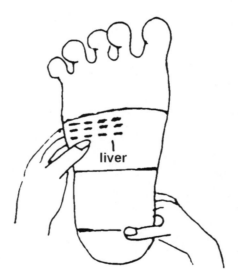

Diagram 2

3. Walk **spine** in both directions three times. Diagram 3.

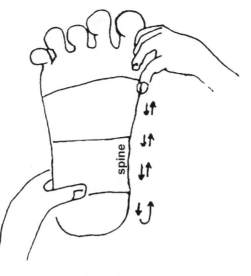

Diagram 3

Repeat exercise 1 and 3 on left foot. Liver is only on right foot.

Now place feet side by side as both feet are worked simultaneously, starting with right foot. Bites must be small and firm and vary according to foot size.

4. Work upwards on **ascending colon** to just beneath the waistline. Between third and fourth toe, turn and walk across onto left foot. Diagram 4.

5. Continue walking across left foot **transverse colon**. Diagram 5.

6. On left foot between third and fourth toe, walk down **descending colon** to heel line. Diagram 6.

7. At heel line, walk back towards right foot and give three presses on **rectum** reflex. Diagram 7.

These diagrams incorporate exercises 4,5,6 and 7

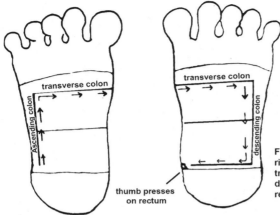

thumb presses
on rectum

For this exercise hold the right foot with right hand and walk ascending and transverse colon with left hand. Walk descending colon and cross left foot to rectum using right hand.

The rectum is a single organ but shown on both feet. The following diagrams explain this. If both feet were joined (at the spine) they'd image the whole body. Therefore an organ either in the front or behind the spine is split into two parts and appear on both feet.

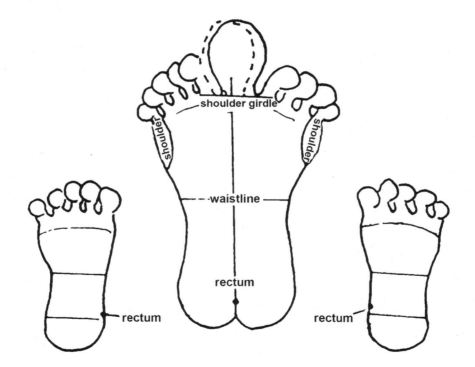

Sciatica This is a most painful condition, caused when the sciatic nerve is inflamed. Pain is felt at back of the thigh and can also affect the lower leg. This condition usually stems from the lower back.

1. Walk down **sciatic** nerve at inner side of leg. Continue across sole of foot, then walk upwards on other side of leg. As leg and feet sizes vary bites will be approximately 30 to 35. Repeat twice. Diagram 1.

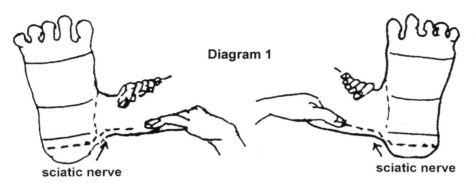

Diagram 1

sciatic nerve   sciatic nerve

The right thumb walks the sciatic nerve on the right leg and across the foot (diagram 1). Then the left hand continues up the latter side of the leg. On the left foot the sequence is started with the left hand working the inner side of the leg and the right hand continues on the latter side.

2. Walk **spine** reflex six times in both directions. Diagram 2.

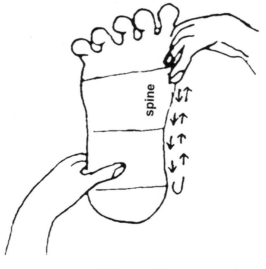

Diagram 2

3. Walk **hip** reflex with five to eight bites and around outer ankle bone. Diagram 3.

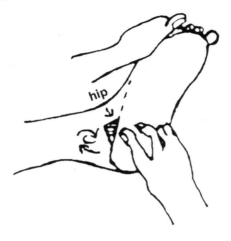

Diagram 3

4. Make three pressure circles on **adrenal** reflex. Diagram 4.

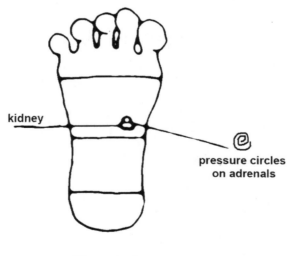

Diagram 4

Repeat on left foot.

Chronic backache This complaint is mega and affects many. Because it's often linked with sciatica these two treatments can be combined. What is the cause? Mainly from lifting something heavy or an awkward twisting movement. The sciatic nerve is 2 cm wide and when inflamed it has a reaction on surrounding tissues, causing severe pain. However, if movement is totally restricted and pain becomes more severe it could indicate a slipped disc, which requires medical attention.

Chronic backache

1. Walk **diaphragm** and give three presses on **solar plexus.** Diagram 1.

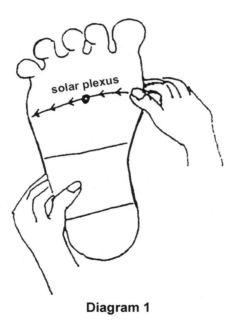

solar plexus

Diagram 1

2. Walk **spine** reflex in alternate directions six times. Diagram 2.

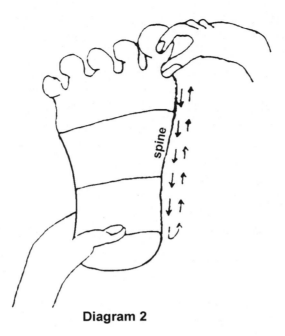

Diagram 2

3.　Make three pressures on **adrenal** reflex. Diagram 3.

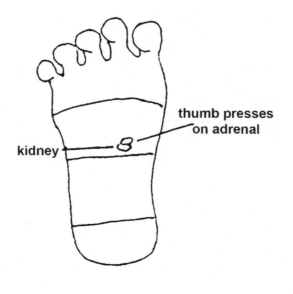

Diagram 3

4. At base of heel, walk upwards to heel line in five to eight lines, working on **gluteals.** The skin on this area is dense, requiring more pressure. Always make sure the side of thumb is used. Diagram 4.

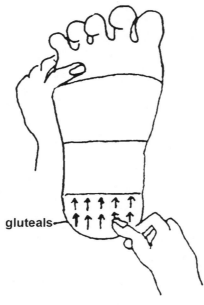

gluteals

Diagram 4

Repeat on left foot.
This condition can be treated two or three times a week.

Tonsillitis Most of us have suffered this at some time or other and know how massively sore the throat feels and even swallowing is difficult. Tonsils are located at the back of the throat and lie either side. They're composed of lymphoid tissue and become inflamed from either viral or bacterial infection.

This has a tremendous impact on the body. Children may have many attacks together with fever and sometimes earache; and then surgery is the only solution.

1. Walk with forefinger across **front of neck** reflex six times. Diagram 1...

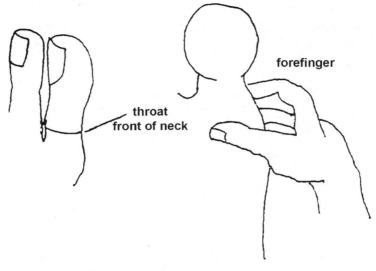

Diagram 1

2. Squeeze **lymphatics** in between toes two to four Diagram 2…

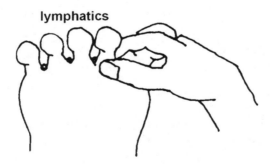

Diagram 2

3. Using forefinger, walk across **lymphatics** (groin) three times ten to thirteen bites. Diagram 3…

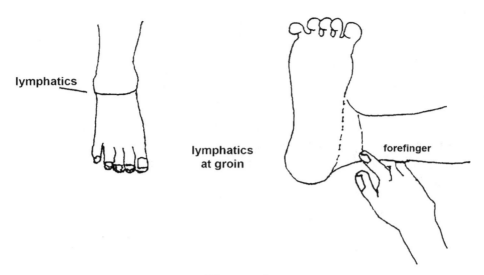

lymphatics

lymphatics
at groin

forefinger

Diagram 3

*Repeat exercises 1, 2, and 3 on left foot, then treat * **spleen** reflex which is <u>on left foot only.</u> See Diagram 4.*

4.   Walk across **spleen** reflex three times seven to eight bites. Diagram 4.

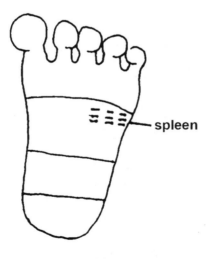

spleen

Diagram 4

This treatment can be done twice a day.

*The spleen is a major part of the immune system where lymphocytes (white blood cells) are found. And these cells are vital in fighting bacteria.

This chapter has explained how foot reflexology embraces the *whole* body and radiates a feeling of well-being. It instils calm even from the beginning when both hands encompass a foot before treatment begins. And there's no reason why babies can't share this too. Their feet are so beautiful and yet so tiny that treatment is mainly massage.

Newborn babies have a lot to contend with. Firstly, their arrival into the world, no longer cocooned in the womb, hearing new sounds and even learning to feed. Therefore it's not surprising babies have long crying periods – sometimes non-stop for three or four hours. Colic is usually to blame. This is associated with trapped wind, which affects one in five babies. Can holding and massaging babies' feet help? Yes it can. But start introducing this early on before those moments of anguish arrive, then having their feet held is associated with comfort.

For these exercises either place baby on a bed, padded table or play-mat.

Colic Only treat centre of sole below fleshy pad underneath toes.

1. Gently hold right foot with left hand, then rock backwards and forwards. Diagram 1.

Every treatment starts with foot holding and rocking as shown in exercise 1

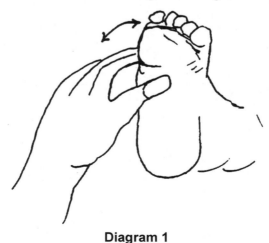

Diagram 1

2. Hold foot with right hand and make 10/12 circles clockwise. Diagram 2.

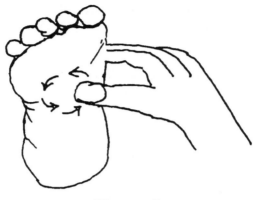

Diagram 2

3. Repeat exercise 1.
4. Work on left foot.

This treats the intestines and can be used for any stomach upsets.

Teething Teething normally happens around five to six months, but like most things with growth and development there's no certainty about this – sometimes earlier or later. But signs give an unmistakeable indication of this: constant drooling, red cheeks, and biting fists. What is, after all, a natural event seems anything but! The following simple exercise helps calm, but again is more successful if learnt before it becomes desperately needed.

1. Start with previous holding and rocking exercise. Diagram 1.

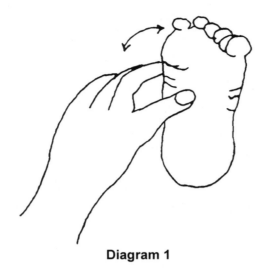

Diagram 1

2. Put right thumb on base of heel and zigzag across foot moving upwards to below toes. Repeat twice. Diagram 2.

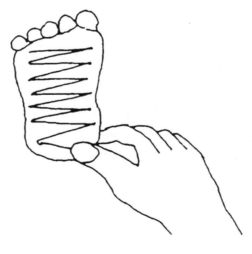

Diagram 2

3. With thumb and forefinger gently squeeze and slide down the front of toes two to five, omitting large toe. Repeat four times. Diagram 3.

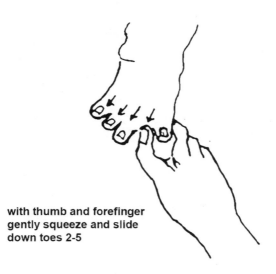

with thumb and forefinger
gently squeeze and slide
down toes 2-5

Diagram 3

4. Finish by repeating exercise 1. Then treat left foot.

<u>Treating Common cold (for babies over four months)</u>

Babies gain more antibodies if they're breastfed which gives immunity to colds and other infections. Today there are many different viruses; and not all are restrained by babies' immunity. This routine is beneficial because it treats the immune system.

1. Start with holding and rocking exercise. Diagram 1.

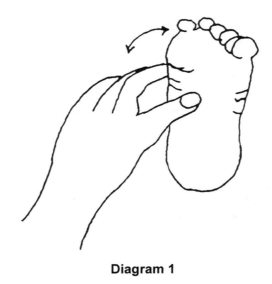

Diagram 1

2. Repeat zigzag movement from previous exercise. Diagram 2.

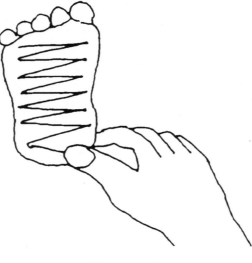

Diagram 2

3. With forefinger, gently press around front of large toe (throat) Do this twice. Diagram 3.

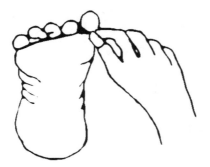

throat at front
of neck

Diagram 3

4. With thumb and forefinger, gently press webbing in between toes. Do this twice. Diagram 4.

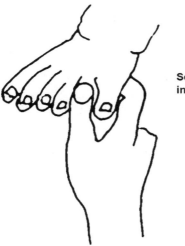

Squeeze webbing
in between toes

Diagram 4

5.   Across ankle crease, make three gentle walks. Then rotate ankle twice. This stimulates the immune system. Diagram 5 & 6.

Work across lymphatics

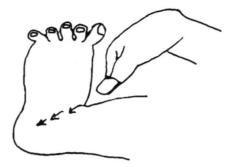

Diagram 5

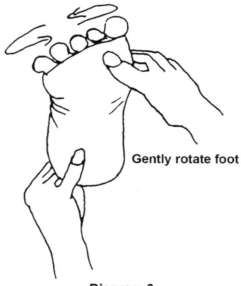

Gently rotate foot

Diagram 6

Repeat on left foot.

This brings baby exercises to an end, which is such a pity because their feet are truly beautiful. But it also means there have been treatments for all the family within this chapter and it gives a good insight into the natural healing of reflexology with a chance to get 'hands on'.

With practice it's possible to know by touch if a reflex feels tight and crunchy even though the recipient says *nothing* – but this is the important feedback needed. Firstly, it confirms the amazing co-ordination between feet and body. Reading about this in print is okay – but when it's your own discovery it confirms that a particular reflex reveals a health problem. This indicates your technique is correct. On the other hand, if someone with acute back or shoulder pain feels no tenderness when the relevant reflexes are pressed, this suggests your technique needs a little more practice. But this is quite understandable when reflexology offers such remarkable challenges to fingers and thumbs.

What is more important is discovering the uniqueness of the holistic approach incorporating mind, body and spirit. This not only creates *wholeness* by putting the body in balance but enables self-healing to take place due to the constant flow of the life-force. With practice treating sensitive reflexes that reveal a blockage in the energy flow, it becomes easier to understand how reflexology works, especially when congestion is removed and the condition improves. This makes practising worthwhile.

These small treatments are adaptable for beginners to practise without causing harm. However it is not advisable to work on the **ovary** and **uterus** reflex for anyone pregnant. An epileptic should not have the head treated. Although reflexology is unlikely to cause a fit should this happen at any time afterwards a wrong conclusion could be reached.

Reflexology is all about natural healing and putting the body in balance, but within this equation lifestyle has to be considered. Smoking, so detrimental to health, is now banned from public places and guidelines from the Food Standards Agency advise eating five portions of fruit and vegetables a day as essential for good health. And following these guidelines helps alleviate serious illness. Food not only fuels the body's energy – the life-force – it too comes under the holistic umbrella. Therefore it's not surprising that accredited reflexology courses include nutrition in their curriculum because it's helpful for some conditions to suggest a natural food remedy in preference to putting chemicals into the body.

Often during treatments the urinary tract is ultra-sensitive. Then advice is given to have a urine sample tested. In the interim cranberry juice is recommended because cranberries have anti-bacterial properties. Even the humble cabbage can treat diarrhoea and sickness, while cinnamon appeases indigestion and bloating.

In the following chapter, 'Food for Thought', food values are clearly put into perspective, with healthy foods on the 'must have' list together with summaries of those to be avoided.

Chapter Six

Food for Thought

Throughout previous chapters there's been continuous reference to the life-force/*chi* circulating through our bodies, but this powerful energy is fuelled by what we eat. A lowered energy reduces the dynamics of the life-force and the body's ability to self-heal. And because of this, a reflexologist asks questions about lifestyle during consultation – relating to smoking, exercise and eating habits. So in this context it's not illogical that reflexology holistically offers the *whole* healthy package which includes advice about natural foods that may benefit a condition.

The Food Standard Agency came into being in 2000 and in the last ten years they have recommended eating five portions of fresh fruit and vegetables a day to avoid serious illness, including cancer. In fact, it's now been established that certain fruit and vegetables can reduce the possibility of having cancer at all. So surely these edibles are destined for the 'must have' list.

Water

This is definitely a 'must have' because water is essential for health. It's always offered after treatment. Why? To remove toxins from the system.

So what are toxins? They're substances that invade the body – pollution from cars, tobacco smoke, and even household refresher sprays. But also when reflexes of the neck, shoulder, and back are treated, small deposits of lactic and uric acid are released which need to be flushed out of the system. Then it's advisable to continue drinking more water at home. The daily recommendation is eight glasses of water a day. And for those falling by the wayside, this is confirmed during treatment when the bladder reflex is pink and puffy from dehydration.

Water forms almost 70 percent of the body and bathes all cells. It's a major component of blood and assists in regulating temperature by sweat excretion.

Water is crucial for life. This has been emphasised when devastating earthquakes have resulted in victims being buried for as long as two weeks but have survived due to finding a small pocket of water. Therefore, even when deprived of food, water can be lifesaving. And a good daily intake improves metabolism which helps weight loss. A question that puzzles most people is whether tap water is preferable to bottled water. Then are there added benefits in opting for carbonated or still? At one time there was controversy regarding the purity of tap water, which encouraged the mineral companies to produce bottled water. However, purifying systems have now been revolutionised, so drinking tap water is safe. In fact some say it has an advantage over bottled types because many fruit-flavoured varieties contain sugar and carbonated water can cause acid reflux which in the long term can affect the oesophagus. Other soft drinks such as soda and diet tonic water also contain sugar. Does this raise concern? Yes it does.

Sugar

This is a carbohydrate destined for the 'garbage bin', because processed sugar has little nutritional value. It creates acidity in the body that affects digestion, causing indigestion and heartburn. But more seriously it causes inflammation that affects joints and arteries. It lowers metabolism and weakens the immune system.

A high sugar intake can result in diabetes, candida or stress whereas natural sugar (fructose) found in whole fruit and vegetables contains vitamins and enzymes beneficial for health. Honey is within this category and is a much better option.

While everyone enjoys the occasional treat, cutting down on sugar really makes sense.

Artificial sweeteners

These are mostly used for tea or coffee because it's assumed they are less fattening than sugar, but they're ten times sweeter and very detrimental to health. These are mainly in fruit juices and many diet drinks, especially those marked 'sugar free', so always read the nutritional advice. Aspartame is a chemical used in many sweeteners marketed under different names; it is so toxic that American air force pilots are not allowed drinks containing it. This is because it can cause many serious health problems, including seizures. Recent reports state if just one small bottle containing a diet fizzy drink is consumed daily the amount of artificial sweeteners it contains increases the risk of diabetes, obesity and heart disease.

Low-calorie drinks command more than 60 percent of the market in the UK, consumed not only by adults but also children. And even though previous studies confirmed these drinks can cause long-term liver damage similar to alcohol abuse, they're still on the market.

But it doesn't end there. Most shoppers know there's sugar in confectionery, cakes, ice cream, puddings and sweet biscuits but it may come as a surprise that it's also in packets of frozen vegetables and convenience packaged meals for microwave cooking, such as 'roast chicken with vegetables', 'shepherd's pie' and 'hake in mornay sauce'. Tinned foods cannot be left out either because there's sugar in soups, including chicken; and again it's in spaghetti, pilchards and baked beans. Popular family snacks such as crisps, garlic bread, pizzas and even the plain cracker succumb to sugar. In the last fifteen years diabetes has *doubled*. Is this surprising?

This suggests that you should always read the nutritional information on all packaged food to make sure the contents are suitable for your diet. But there are so many different foods and beverages that have amazing healing properties, such as green tea. But who would expect drinking a 'cuppa' could protect the body in so many ways? Frequently reflexology is sought after by those suffering fatigue and constantly plagued by colds and other viruses. And what do the foot reflexes reveal? The whole immune system weakened; which means the life-force is depleted, and this lack of energy is not strong enough to combat the invasion of bacteria and viruses. Reflexologists then treat these specific reflexes – but also suggest green tea. Not especially a breakfast drink, more preferable in the afternoon. And opt for pure green tea rather than mixed varieties. Instructions advise that you should always make it with water just below boiling point.

Green tea

Numerous studies have identified green tea as anti-viral, anti-inflammatory, and anti-microbial, making it a wonderful panacea against colds and influenza. It also inhibits histamines and has diuretic functions. Recent tests by cancer experts show it has anti-cancer properties that slow down the growth of cancer cells. Put this on the 'must have' list.

Arthritis afflicts 20 million people in the UK. These numbers refer to osteoarthritis when it's advised to cut down on acidic foods such as red meat and dairy products. But as we already know not drinking enough water and excess sugar can exacerbate inflammation in the body. Discovering that food can have this effect on our systems may be just as surprising as finding out about foods that can help. Cutting down on dairy can pose a dilemma.

But soya milk is an excellent alternative. Ginger, too, reduces inflammation in the body. Rather than buying it in supplement form, chopped ginger can be cooked with stewed apple: a delicious extra for breakfast with cereal.

Soya

Soya bean products include milk, tofu – which is used as an alternative to meat dishes such as mince and sausages – and edamame soya beans can be bought as frozen vegetables. Apart from being a good milk alternative, studies in New York show soya helps reduce breast cancer in women and inhibits prostate cancer cells spreading in men. But what are the compounds in soya that enable this to happen? They're called isoflavones and in structure similar to the female hormone oestrogen. It's during the menopause that the level of oestrogen drops. This causes night sweats and hot flushes.

In Japan where more soya is eaten 'hot flushes' are unheard of. They also have fewer cases of high cholesterol, heart disease and breast cancer. So experiment: soya mince can be used in cottage pie, spaghetti Bolognese or chilli con carne.

Today figures show levels of heart disease in the UK have risen to more than 152,000. Statins are prescribed to reduce blood pressure; but reflexology is able to do this. Once again this is due to the principle of reflexology that creates balance and harmony in the body. This means that a high level of blood pressure is lowered and low blood pressure is increased, rather like the balancing act of a pair of scales. But what causes high blood pressure?

Salt – sodium chloride

The body needs salt to exist, but too much salt causes high blood pressure. Salt levels in the body are controlled by the kidneys, but if salt exceeds the amount kidneys are able to control it leaks into the bloodstream. This attracts water which increases the volume of blood and raises blood pressure. Then there is more possibility of cardiovascular disease, strokes and kidney failure.

Recommendation for salt intake is one level teaspoonful or 6 grams a day for an adult. Alternatives are mineral rock salt or low sodium salt. Once again, diet food falls by the wayside: one make of diet crisps has 6 grams of salt in a 16 gram packet! – one whole day's salt requirement. This underlines the need to read all food labels.

High cholesterol levels can also cause hypertension and strokes. Yet our bodies need it for cells' sustenance. It circulates in the bloodstream attached to two different proteins. HDL (high density protein) carries 'good' cholesterol in the bloodstream to the liver where it's synthesised. But then there's the 'bad guy' – LDL (low density lipoprotein) – which deposits debris in arteries that not only narrows them but ultimately causes blockages and serious heart disease. Although high cholesterol can be genetic it's mainly down to eating too much saturated fat, processed food, and high energy foods like red meat, smoking, and restricted intake of fresh fruit and vegetables. The exact reason why the Food Standards Agency have promoted 'eat five a day' is because scientists have been testing the healing properties of various fruits and vegetables for years and know that *natural* is better than processed food or drinks with additives.

Now we know that antioxidants contained in certain foods and beverages (such as green tea) protect against cancer. Antioxidants are substances that neutralise free radicals in the body (toxins) which can damage and change cell tissue. These toxins have the ability to distort DNA, attack blood vessels and damage brain cells. But antioxidants protect and defend the body from free radical damage which includes cancer. The good news is that many *foods* contain antioxidant enzymes, putting the body in balance without chemicals, which takes us back to homeostatis.

The purpose of this chapter has been to summarise what's good and what's bad in a diet and how this affects the body. It's also meant that some items have been assigned to the garbage bin because they cause health issues, such as sugar, artificial sweeteners, and salt. Patients with hypertension or high cholesterol are prescribed statins. This medication is still under scrutiny because recent allegations suggest it's being over-prescribed, meaning that almost 40 percent of patients need not be on them at all. Perhaps it's time to think more about what fresh foods have to offer because they provide an amazing abundance of *natural* medicine.

Both potassium and magnesium are found in various fresh fruits, nuts, whole grains, vegetables, poultry, seafood and yoghurt. Both these minerals have a profound impact on the heart. Potassium acts on nerve impulses for muscle contraction and regulates both heartbeat and blood pressure. Magnesium also reduces blood pressure, inhibits blood clots (warding off strokes) and widens arteries. Then together with potassium it regulates heart rhythms. There is no end to this mineral's versatility because it also reduces cholesterol.

What vegetables can be eaten to lower high blood pressure? A wide variety: broccoli, spinach, cabbage, carrots, swede, potatoes, peppers, peas, beetroot, Brussels sprouts, watercress, tomatoes, parsley and garlic. But beetroot must have a special mention because it's a high performer in reducing blood pressure by widening blood vessels. Its impact on reducing heart disease is considerable; so much so that tests have been carried out on beetroot juice and it is now available in health shops. Researchers at Queen Mary University of London compared some patients drinking 250 ml glasses of juice with those taking nitrate tablets. The result – the same! Drinking just one glass of beetroot juice a day lowers blood pressure in 24 hours; for those suffering hypertension, then, this is definitely for the 'must have' list. There is just one colourful side-effect – purple pee!

Bananas, too, have a high potassium content, making them a good start for the day if eaten at breakfast. Other fruits containing this mineral are oranges, grapefruit, pineapple, peaches, cantaloupe melon, apples, blackberries, strawberries, kiwi fruit, avocado pears and dates. Most fruits are eaten fresh, which maintains potassium content; if boiled, potassium levels in food is lowered, therefore it's better to cook by either microwave or steam.

Some fruit and vegetables contain not only potassium and magnesium but also antioxidants, which are said to inhibit cancer.

A diet low in magnesium is mostly due to diet and is recommended for patients with fibromyalgia who find that reflexology helps their condition. They suffer fatigue from constant pain throughout the body, and also insomnia. Magnesium fights fatigue and aids muscle relaxation which removes tension and cramps. This mineral is found in the following foods.

Nuts are a good source, particularly almonds, cashew, walnuts, and Brazil nuts. The fat in nuts is mono-unsaturated, so small amounts do not cause weight problems and eating just seven walnuts a day reduces cholesterol. At Marshall University in West Virginia researchers found that walnuts protect against breast cancer. What an astounding bevy of 'must haves' in a nutshell!

Magnesium can be found in: all green leafy vegetables, as well as celery; legumes, such as kidney, lima and soy beans and lentils; unprocessed 'breakfast' grains like oats and bran, as well as wild and brown rice; fruits like bananas, grapes, avocados, blackberries, raspberries and watermelon; fish, including salmon and halibut. Always tired? Magnesium can help.

But for a healthy heart Omega-3 essential acids cannot be ignored, and The British Heart Foundation recommend eating two portions of fish a week, particularly oily fish such as salmon, mackerel, herring, tuna and sardines for maximum benefit. In Japan and Greenland, where more fish is eaten, there are lower rates of strokes and heart disease.

So far the focus has been looking at foods that help prevent these conditions and some that lower the risk of cancer. The latest statistics for the UK show that one in three people will be diagnosed with cancer in their lifetime. This is horrendous when it's believed this figure could be less if more people ate fresh food rather than processed, stopped smoking and reduced alcohol intake.

Sadly, any condition already manifested in the body cannot be healed by reflexology, but patients who have treatments find it helps reduce the after effects of chemotherapy, and feel more assured with a strong resilience of purpose. Many foods and some beverages are said to protect and inhibit cancer, but how? The answer relates to the antioxidants made up from different enzymes which include beta carotene, and some vitamins including A, C and E. So once again it comes back to having the right diet with plenty of antioxidants able to protect and defend the body against free radicals that change cell formation. Many of the fruits and vegetables already mentioned are bursting with these components able to do this, but some foods are especially accredited to specific cancers such as bladder cancer (causing 7,646 deaths a year in the UK) and scientists at Ohio State University say 'eating broccoli can restrict its spread'. Scientists at the University of California also maintain cruciferous vegetables – cauliflower, broccoli and cabbage – 'inhibit rapid growth of tumour cells in breast cancer in a similar way to chemotherapy'. Deaths from breast cancer in the UK amount to 48,450. These figures are alarming. However, there is some good news for coffee drinkers because at the National Cancer Centre in Tokyo scientists state that coffee drinkers (restricted to two cups a day) are 42 percent less likely to have liver cancer than non-coffee drinkers. This conclusion was reached after more than 60,000 people were studied over a nine-year period.

Most berries are high in beta carotene protecting against this disease, such as blueberries, strawberries, raspberries and blackberries. It's also found in the lush yellow, red and orange fruits and vegetables. Here we're looking at peppers, sweet potatoes, butternut squash, carrots, oranges, apricots, tomatoes and cantaloupe melon.

The 'Mediterranean diet' is said to be healthy because olive oil is widely used, together with tomatoes, garlic and mixed salads. All these items are fresh natural foods that have anti-cancer properties. A number of doctors subscribe to the overwhelming importance of diet for good health, such as Dr Andrew Weil MD, who has written many books about natural food protecting the body's healing system and regards himself as a mind/body practitioner. This approach follows the holistic path where evaluation of reflexology relates to the body's ability to self-heal by enhancing the flow of the life-force. This dynamic energy flowing through our bodies promotes healing. But this natural energy – the life-force – needs power to be effective which can only come from eating healthy food. It's this combination that contributes to *natural healing with reflexology.*

Footnotes

During a lifetime the average person walks 115,000 miles. Therefore it's not unusual that some of the following foot problems have been experienced.

Athlete's foot is a fungal disease often picked up either at swimming pools or gyms. It is very contagious. Because of this wear your own flip-flops instead of walking barefoot. How is it detected? The skin appears damp and soggy, with itchy patches of skin in between the toes. The skin may crack, bleed or flake and have a pungent odour.

Treatment is by over-the-counter ointment from chemists. Keep feet dry, preferably using paper towels; never share towels and wear cotton socks. Also cut down on sugar intake.

Bunion is caused by a joint deficiency at the hallux (large toe). This pushes the large toe inwards towards the other toes. This causes a bursa (sac containing fluid) to develop over the bony prominence as protection. Inflammation ensues and a hard lump develops. This can be a painful condition requiring surgery. Major cause of this condition is due to 'killer heels' or squashing feet into tight shoes.

Corns are divided into three varieties – hard, soft and seed. Hard corns appear on yellowish patches of hard skin due to abnormal pressure. The soft variety form in between toes caused by pressure and sweat. Seed corns are minute, the size of a pinhead and exist in dry skin. Corns can be removed with corn plasters, or treated by a podiatrist. Keep feet healthy by removing hard skin and moisturise.

Calluses are often found on pressure points and bony parts of toes, and are usually due to ill-fitting shoes. After soaking feet, use a foot-scraper to remove hard skin. However, diabetic patients (often through nerve damage) have numbness in their feet and cannot always feel something sharp. Because of this they may be unaware of skin abrasion which could cause serious implications. Therefore diabetics should have their feet treated by a podiatrist.

Chilblains occur in wintertime. Sufferers usually have poor circulation and need to keep feet warmly covered. Toes become pink and swollen, itch and sometimes crack. Feet that are massively cold should not be warmed quickly by direct heat – electric fire or hot water bottle. Chilblains are not solely confined to feet but can be seen on ears and backs of legs. Scratching causes skin abrasion and possible infection. Ointments are available at chemists.

Fungal nail infection is caused by the same fungus as athlete's foot. Nails thicken and change colour, and part of the nail may crumble. Without treatment it worsens and infects other nails. Medical treatment is necessary and a doctor will send clippings away for analysis. Sometimes the nails need to be painted with an anti-fungal nail paint which needs two applications a week. Also anti-fungal tablets are prescribed. Recovery time? Six months or even a year.

Ganglion is a benign cyst seen on dorsal (front) of foot. It is not usually painful unless pressing on nerves, when it may need to be surgically removed. Years ago this was done by a doctor whamming down on the cyst with a huge book to disperse it – and it worked!

Gout is caused by an excess of uric acid. Usually it affects the large toe that swells and becomes extremely painful – even affecting walking. This condition is due to diet. Therefore omit eating acidic foods such as meat, cheese, rhubarb, oranges and beer. All are main contributors to uric acid formation. Gout not only affects feet but also elbows and knees. Medication can be prescribed.

Ingrowing toenails usually affects the large toe and is caused through incorrectly cutting the nail. This should be cut straight across, not too short and without sharp edges that can pierce the skin. This causes infection and pus. The area must be kept clean and soaking in salt water draws out impurities. If the infection does not improve, seek doctor's advice.

Metatarsalgia is a painful condition, often caused from wearing high heels when acute pressure is put on the ball of the foot causing a build-up of hard skin beneath the toes. This condition is also prevalent in runners wearing inappropriate footwear for use on hard surfaces.

The pressure affects and distorts the metatarsal bones. A podiatrist can manipulate bones to ease pain.

Morton's neuroma is due to an enlarged nerve usually between third and fourth toe. And although 'neuroma' means tumour, here it means nerve enlargement. Mostly the nerve between the third and fourth toe is affected, causing pain and numbness in these toes. How does this happen? Through injury, sport or tight-fitting shoes. Steroid injections can be given, or the last resort is to have the nerve removed surgically.

Plantar fasciitis is heel pain and was once called 'policeman's foot'. Pain is caused when the plantar fascia which supports the arch becomes inflamed. This causes sharp stabbing pain at the heel and movement is restricted because the arch is unable to lift and spring. Sometimes the tendon calcifies and creates a spur. Cortisone may be given or local anaesthetic injected at the heel to remove both pain and inflammation.

Smelly feet can be caused from footwear not allowing the foot to breathe, particularly those made from synthetic material. This creates interaction between perspiration and bacteria that generates the smell. Excessive perspiration can be due to stress, medication, or spicy food. Bathe feet regularly in tepid water, wear cotton or wool socks. Change shoes every two days. Insert charcoal in-soles. Use anti-foot odour powders or sprays to deodorise feet. Alternatively soak feet in strong black tea for 30 minutes twice a week: the tannic acid kills bacteria and closes pores. Remedy: two teabags per pint of water; boil for 15 minutes then add two quarts of cool water. Soak feet for 30 minutes.

Verrucae are flat warts and are viral. They are very contagious. Skin around a verruca is raised and whitish with a dark brown/black centre. Once identified, cover with plaster to stop the spread. How can it be removed? A podiatrist might use a freezing technique or there are removal solutions at chemists. A home remedy is to tape over the verruca with the inner side of banana skin. Change this daily. Remarkably, it works.

USEFUL ADDRESSES

International Institute of Reflexology.
Head Office 3 Ashley Lane Killamarsh, Sheffield
National Director: Vicky Laws
Tel.no. 0114 247 1725
Email Vicky@reflexology-uk.net

The International Federation of Reflexologists,
8-9 Talbot Court London EC3V OBP
Tel.no. 0870 3562
www.intfedreflexology.org.

Lynne Booth VRT Courses
Booth VRT Limited Suite 205
60 Westbury Hill Bristol BS9 JUJ
Tel.no. + 44 (0) 1179 626746
Email: contact@boothvrt.com

Association of Reflexology
5 Fore Street
Taunton
Somerset
Tel.no.01823 351010